THE
GENIUS OF HOMOEOPATHY

LECTUERS AND ESSAYS
ON
HOMOEOPATHIC PHILOSOPHY

By

STUART CLOSE, M.D.

*Late Professor of Homoeopathic Philosophy,
New York Homoeopathic Medical College and Flower Hospital;
Editor, Department of Homoepathic Philosophy of The Homoeopathic
Recorder; Consulting Physician, Prospect Heights Hospital, Brooklyn, N.Y.;
Member, American Institute of Homoeopathy; Member, Ex-President and
Senior, International Hahnemannian Association; Member, Kings County
Medical Society; Founder, Brooklyn Hahnemannian Union; Member
National, New York State and Long Island Historical Associations;
Advisor, American Foundation for Homoeopathy, etc.*

B. JAIN PUBLISHERS PVT. LTD.
NEW DELHI - 110 055

Price : Rs. 25.00

Reptint Edition : 1993

© Copyright with the Publisher

Published by :
B. Jain Publishers Pvt. Ltd.
1921, Street No. 10, Chuna Mandi
Paharganj, New Delhi - 110 055 (INDIA)

Printed at :
J.J. Offset Printers
Kishan Kunj, Delhi - 110 092
ISBN 81-7021-108-5
BOOK CODE B-2167

DEDICATED
TO THE MEMORY OF MY REVERED PRECEPTORS
PHINEAS PARKHURST WELLS, M. D.
(1808-1891)

AND

BERNHARDT FINCKE, M. D.
(1821-1906)
TRUE FRIENDS, GREAT PHYSICIANS,
PROFOUND PHILOSOPHERS AND LOYAL FOLLOWERS

OF

SAMUEL HAHNEMANN

PREFACE

MANY of the articles which make up this book were originally prepared and delivered as lectures for the Senior Classes of the New York Homœopathic Medical College, during my engagement as Professor of Homœopathic Philosophy, 1909-1913. Most of them, after revision, have appeared during the past four years in the Department of Homœopathic Philosophy conducted by me in The Homœopathic Recorder. Revised again, they are now issued in compliance with many requests from readers of The Recorder and others, who have expressed their belief that they are worthy of preservation and that their publication in book form will serve a useful purpose.

In discussing Hahnemannian principles from a modern standpoint I hope to contribute something toward a renewal of interest in the science and art of therapeutic medication as exemplified in Homœopathy, of which the medical profession is much in need.

A review of current literature and neighborly relations with many physicians of the dominant school of medicine reveals not only a more friendly spirit than formerly existed, but an active interest in what their homœopathic brethren have to offer toward the solution of therapeutic problems and a desire to co-operate. The era of therapeutic nihilism is passing away. Thinking men and leaders of the dominant school are ready to participate in a scientific discussion of the theory and principles of therapeutic medication from a homœopathic standpoint when approached in a non-sectarian spirit. They are becoming more generally receptive of the idea of the existence of a general principle or law of therapeutic medication than ever before and more willing to consider evidence submitted in favor of that proposition. They rightly hold, however, that the evidence to be submitted should be prepared in such a manner as to comply with the requirements of scientific research. Leaving that phase of the subject to the scientific and research workers and others to whom it may be congenial, and not forgetting the many in our own school who are interested, it seems permissible to present once more, as simply and attractively as possible, an exposition of the logical, historical and philosophical principles upon which Homœopathy is based and attempt to show, at least suggestively, its relation as a department of general medicine to other sciences. That is the object of this book. It makes no pretensions to being "scientific." It is conceived and submitted in a fraternal and philosophic spirit, however far it may fall short of adequate expression.

STUART CLOSE.

Brooklyn, N. Y.

CONTENTS

Chapter		Page
	Dedication	
	Preface	
I.	The Psychological Point of View	1
II.	General Interpretations	8
III.	Schools of Philosophy	23
IV.	The Scope of Homœopathy	37
V.	The Unity of Medicine	48
VI.	Life, Health and Disease	60
VII.	Susceptibility, Reaction and Immunity	76
VIII.	General Pathology of Homœopathy	87
IX.	Cure and Recovery	122
X.	Indisposition and the Second Best Remedy	135
XI.	Symptomatology	147
XII.	Examination of the Patient	167
XIII.	Homœopathic Posology	183
XIV.	Potentiation and the Infinitesimal Dose	212
XV.	The Drug Potential	237
XVI.	The Logic of Homœopathy	244
XVII.	The Development of Hahnemannian Philosophy in the Sixth Edition of The Organon	271
	Index	275

INTRODUCTION

CHAPTER I

The Psychological Point of View

Great Personalities.—All great forward movements in religion, science or art originate in the mind of some individual who appears at the psychological moment and announces his mission. His personality and his teaching represent the truth for which he stands.

To a Moses or a Luther, to a Washington or a Lincoln, to a Plato or a Bacon, to a Hippocrates or a Hahnemann, each in his own sphere and period, the world comes and must come for instruction, inspiration and leadership.

Always, following the appearance of a great teacher or leader, opponents, detractors, or corruptors spring up and attempt to stay, or destroy, or divert to their own glory the progress of the new movement. Disciples or would-be disciples have always to be on guard against false teaching. Their principal safeguard is in maintaining a sincere and intelligent loyalty to the historic leader whose personality and teachings represent the original truth, and in intellectual and personal fellowship with other followers who maintain the same attitude and relation.

Lesser lights and lesser leaders there must and always will be, to whom, each in his own rank and degree, honor and loyalty are due; but the disciple is never above his master. He only is "The Master" to whom the first great revelation of truth was made and by whom it was first developed and proclaimed; for such epochal men are supremely endowed and specially prepared, usually by many years of seclusion, intense thought and labor. They are raised up at last to do a great work. They stand on the mountain tops of human experience, from whence they have a field of view and a grasp of truth never before attainable. Like

Moses they have, as it were, received the "Tables of the Law" direct from the hand of the Almighty.

Homœopathy, the science and art of therapeutic medication, has a twofold existence—as an institution and in the personnel of its loyal, individual representatives.

These two constituents are pervaded by a common animating spirit, which finds expression respectively in its organizations and literature and in the life and practice of its followers.

Homœopathy a System.—The fundamental principles of homœopathy are embodied in a system of doctrines, laws and rules of practice which were first formulated, named and systematically set forth by Hahnemann in his Organon of the Rational Art of Healing. By that, homœopathy was given a name, an individuality and a character which defines and identifies it for all time.

The practical demonstration of homœopathy is committed to its personal representatives, whose success will be proportionate to their efficiency. Efficiency in homœopathy implies and involves native ability, acquired technical proficiency and logical consistency in the application of its principles. The exercise of these qualifications requires honesty, courage, fidelity to a high ideal and a right point of view.

Every problem with which homœopathy deals, therefore, must be approached and every technical process conducted systematically from a particular and definite mental standpoint. The student or practitioner of homœopathy must not only know what this point of view is, but he must acquire it and act from it in each case. This might be called the personal side of homœopathy; for in the last analysis homœopathy, from the psychological standpoint, is essentially a state of mind existent in the person of its representative. In this sense personality, or the sum of all the essential attributes and qualities of the individual is a condition-precedent to professional success.

Having defined the qualities and attributes that enter into the make-up of the homœopathician the various practical problems and technical processes of homœopathy can be taken up and discussed from the point of view already established.

As a prerequisite to a clear understanding of the subject,

as well as to the attainment of efficiency in the practical application of its principles, it is assumed that homœopathy is what it is claimed to be, a complete system of therapeutic medication. As a scientific system it is made up of certain facts, laws, rules and methods or processes, each of which is an integral part of the whole.

Nothing conflicting with its established principles can be added to it, nothing taken away, if it is to stand in its integrity. Once it is determined what these essential elements and principles are, homœopathy must stand or fall as a whole.

A mutilated homœopathy is a lame and crippled thing, compelled to sustain itself by crutches, splints and braces. An emasculated homœopathy is an impotent homœopathy, without the virility necessary to maintain or reproduce itself. Some short-sighted, superficial and weak-kneed individuals, actuated by their prejudices, or through their failure to comprehend the subject as a whole, have adopted an emasculated homœopathy for themselves and attempted to support their crippled eunuch as a candidate for general acceptance. Subjects such as the "life force" the single remedy, potentiation, infinitesimals, the minimum dose, and the totality of the symptoms as a basis for the prescription, they have characterized as unessential, "so long as the principle of *similia* was maintained." They do not perceive that each of these doctrines is logically drawn from and inseparably connected with the one fundamental doctrine which they profess to accept and apply. It is this which has brought homœopathy, *as an institution,* down to a point where its very existence is threatened.

Within its sphere homœopathy is entirely adequate to meet all its own problems in its own way, when it is practiced in its purity and entirety. But homœopathy will fail if it is forced outside or beyond its real sphere, or if it is perverted and emasculated. To know the true sphere and limitations of homœopathy is as necessary to practical success as to know its technic and resources.

Mere formal knowledge of the "law of cure" and the technic of prescribing does not make a homœopathic physician in the **true** sense of the word. Something more than that is needed. **Into that cold and inert body the breath of life must be breathed** before it becomes a living soul. Homœopathy is a spirit as well as a body of rules and principles and the spirit must be incarnated in every true believer and follower. That incarnation takes place when the mind of the neophyte is opened to the philosophical truths which underlie both the method and the principles, and he becomes imbued with the desire and the purpose to make them the ruling influence of his life.

Methods of adapting and applying the principles have changed to some extent as the scope and technic of prescribing have been developed, but homœopathy is essentially the same to-day that it was a hundred years ago. Individual practitioners, nominally followers of Hahnemann, have drifted away from his teachings and method, and some have attempted to inject into or graft upon homœopathy all sorts of "fads and fancies;" but the mongrel thing thereby created deceives no one who has derived his knowledge from the fountain head. Homœopathy as set forth by Hahnemann, while not perfect, is complete in all essentials as a system. It is supreme within its legitimate sphere because it is the only method of therapeutic medication which is based upon a fixed and definite law of nature.

The validity of this law has been disputed by the dominant school of medicine ever since it was first promulgated by Hahnemann; but it has never been denied by any one who has complied with all the conditions necessary for a scientific demonstration of its verity. To comply with those conditions in good faith and test the matter is to be convinced.

It is conceivable and probably true that one reason for the rejection of the homœopathic principle is that the principle, as usually stated, has never been fully understood. It is a fact that most, if not all of the attempts (with an exception to be brought forward later) to state the principle have been faulty. Analysis and comparison have not been carried far enough, in most cases, to clearly identify the principle and its relations, and establish homœopathy in the "circle of the sciences" where it belongs.

The dominant school of medicine has not only denied that the so-called "homœopathic law" is a law of nature, but denied that there is any general law which governs the relation between drugs and disease and have ceased searching for one. The existing situation has never been better characterized than by Mons. Marchand de Calvi in an eloquent and stirring address to the French Academy of Medicine.

"In medicine," he said, "there is not, nor has there been for some time, either principle, faith or law. We build a Tower of Babel, or rather we are not so far advanced, for we build nothing; we are in a vast plain where a multitude of people pass backwards and forwards; some carry bricks, others pebbles, others grains of sand, but no one dreams of *the cement;* the foundations of the edifice are not yet laid, and as to the general plan of the work, it is not even sketched. In other words, medical literature swarms with facts, of which the most part are periodically produced with the most tiresome monotony; these are called observations and clinical facts; a number of laborers consider and reconsider particular questions of pathology or therapeutics—that is called original research. The mass of such labors and facts is enormous; no reader can wade through them—but no one has any general doctrine. The most general doctrine that exists is the *doctrine of homœopathy!* This is strange and lamentable; a disgrace to medicine—but—such is the fact."

Principles and Organizations.—A common mistake, and one of the greatest that can be made, is that of rendering to organizations the spiritual submission that belongs in the highest degree to principles only.

Organizations are formed for the purpose of maintaining and advancing principles, but it often happens that in the stress of building and maintaining the organization the principles are pushed into the background, neglected or forgotten. The man too often becomes the slave of the machine instead of its master. The organization becomes a Frankenstein which destroys its creator. Worse even than the mere neglect or forgetting, is the wilful corruption and perversion of principles which is often the result of the mad struggle for organization prestige, power and position. Moreover, individuals connected with or responsible for the success of the organization are easily infected with the germ of selfish personal ambition. They come to regard their official contract with it as a through ticket on The Limited to the city of their dreams.

Out of these conditions, which it is not necessary to illustrate or enlarge upon, arise some of the most serious problems of the world. Organizations—civil, military, medical, political, social, religious and educational—may and often do become corrupt, mercenary, tyrannical; a menace to liberty and progress; enemies to the principles they are supposed to represent and agents of compulsion.

The individual truth-seeker must, therefore, keep his eyes open and walk circumspectly if he would keep in the path of progress, maintain his mental integrity and preserve liberty of thought, speech and action.

It has come to pass that individual liberty is calculated only in percentages now. The increasing pressure of official and institutional compulsion encircles us. The moral compulsion of the "Drive" is but a short remove from the physical compulsion of the "Draft." Metaphorically, the internment camp, the prison, the dead wall and the firing squad are just beyond.

The world is in a state of war. It is a "War of the Worlds." The political world, the industrial world, the social world, the religious world, the medical world—organizations all—are torn by war because importance has been attached to organizations that belongs only to principles.

Organizations like men are subject to disease, decay and death. When they become corrupt they die, for corruption is elementary death. Institutions, nations, whole civilizations have died, disappeared and been forgotten until brought to light by the excavations of archeologists centuries or perhaps millenniums afterwards. But principles never die.

Principles are essential truth, represented by or corresponding to facts. The essential characteristic of truth is its steadfast conformity to law and order. Truth is Life, Mind, Spirit; absolute, infinite and immortal. Organisms in which truth embodies itself are transitory. They change, decay and pass away, but life is continuous. Truth, like the fabled Phœnix, burns itself on the altar and arises from its own ashes.

Homœopathy, as already pointed out, has a two-fold existence—as an institution or organization and in the individuals who make up its following. The spirit and principles of homœopathy have never been and never can be solely in the keeping of any institution, for organizations are continually changing and dying.

Individuals unite in small or great societies and work together harmoniously for a time, but not for long. Disagreements arise, they dissolve their original relations and form others; but the work goes on because the Spirit of Truth always draws together those of like minds for the attainment of a common object. At critical periods and in the long run it is always the individual who preserves, passes on and perpetuates the truth.

Upon individuals, therefore, as living embodiments and representatives of the truth, rests a great and solemn responsibility. No man can shift his personal responsibility to an organization. As a creator and member of organizations he does not cease to be an individual trustee, nor should he become slavishly subject to the organization. The creator is greater than the creature. He may work in or by means of an organization, but he may not work for an organization, lest he presently find himself in bondage to a creature which has become corrupt.

It follows that our greatest concern as followers of Hahnemann and representatives of homœopathy is primarily with individuals—with men and principles rather than with organizations. We will build men into organizations and keep the organizations clean and useful as well and as long as we can; but let us be sure that we *build principles into men.*

Nature puts man first. Truth is not revealed to institutions, but to men. Let us have done with fictions and deal with realities. An organization is a machine; an inanimate, soulless thing; a figment of the imagination; a creature of the law, deriving its existence and seeming vitality only from the individual men who compose it; ceasing to be when their relations are dissolved. Man is a real living, thinking human being, "made in the image and likeness of God," an individual embodiment and personification of a portion of the Infinite and Universal Mind, endowed with the ability to exercise creative power within his appointed sphere and destined for immortality. Let him exercise it in liberty, using organizations judiciously but not becoming enslaved by them.

CHAPTER II

General Interpretations

The Philosophy of Homœopathy rests upon the following general interpretations of the System of Nature which Science universally recognizes as fundamental.
1. The laws and ways of Nature are uniform and harmonious.
2. Effects follow causes in unbroken succession.
3. To every action there is an equal and opposite reaction.
4. Action and reaction are ceaseless, equivalent and reciprocal
5. Motion is ceaseless and transformation continuous.
6. Matter is indestructible and infinitely divisible.
7. Force is persistent and indestructible.
8. The quantity of action necessary to effect any change in nature is the least possible.

The following propositions, slightly modified from the original, are drawn from Von Grauvogl's Text Book of Homœopathy. (Nuremburg, 1865; London, New York and Chicago, 1870. Trans. by George E. Shipman, M. D.)

The aim of all science is to set up in place of the *contingent* that which law makes *necessary,* and to refer every particular to its universal.

These two predicates connect science with things.

We must hold fast intellectually to the useful things which the past has produced. We must gain *space* in *time,* but *living space.* Not by the empiric accumulation of facts *perceived* (the facts of perception), but by their well weighed *appreciation,* according to the eternal laws of nature, is their existence secured for all time. Facts which this criterion rejects are worthless scientifically.

Hence in homœopathy we strive not only to separate the contingency from the event, *i. e.,* to determine the causal succession from what has taken place, but also to become master of that contingency which makes our judgment uncertain. The contingency of our judgment of the facts, arrived at experimentally by the process of analysis, must be removed synthetically by connecting the laws of nature with the facts, so that we may be able to show their interdependence and act accordingly. In this synthesis, or connecting of our perceptions, conducted simultaneously with experimentation, consists *the Art of observation.*

All conceptions of our inner being, as well as external things, are based primarily upon the perceptions of our senses (including consciousness, or the "inner sense"). But the formation of our ideas, judgments and conclusions must result from determinate, objective laws, inherent in the things themselves and their constitution, and not from caprice.

Every event in the circle of natural phenomena has a *conditional* necessity, since it can only result from its precedents and depends upon them. This conditional necessity results from the primary *unconditional* necessity of the fundamental laws of nature and their absolute truth.

Laws of nature are the forms by which the constant course of natural phenomena from given causes and conditions may be expressed.

Laws do not cause the *existence* of events or phenomena. By virtue of the laws we may explain to ourselves, intellectually, not the *existence,* but the *connection* of phenomena, and so come to understand their development and conditions.

We understand phenomena, not by any apparent properties of the phenomena themselves, but by intuitive perception or immediate consciousness of the fundamental laws. Such laws as the law of cause and effect, the equivalence and contrariety of action and reaction, the constancy of matter and force, are intuitively perceived to be the ultimate reason of which we can have any knowledge.

Laws of nature, in general, are deductions of experience and observations with regard to the necessary course of events or phenomena from given elements, the ultimate course of which lies beyond physical science in the domain of metaphysics.

That which *changes* the regular course of states and events, however, results in consequence of causes which may be determined by physical science by considering the fundamental laws of nature.

Every change of state or event has a number of causes, known as primary and secondary causes, or as cause and conditions.

A spark of fire, put into a barrel of powder, is the *cause* of the explosion that follows. The chemical composition of the constitutents of the powder and their mode of combination supply the necessary *conditions* for explosion to occur.

Every *change* implies or presupposes something *constant,* that is, something with at least two opposite tendencies. Chemistry, *e. g.,* rests upon the law of constancy of bodies and forces, the law of chemical affinity and the law of definite proportions or equivalence.

In accordance with the law of constancy of bodies and forces, all bodies remain essentially the same under all circumstances. Chlorine remains chlorine, and hydrogen remains hydrogen always. Only as they are combined according to the laws of chemical affinity, and certain definite proportions, do they change *their state* and become hydrochloric acid. The *cause* of this result lies in the art of the chemist. The *conditions* lie in the specific affinity of these bodies for each other and for other bodies. The *effect* is to change their two states into one in the form of hydrochloric acid.

The *cause* of tuberculosis is the tubercle bacillus.

The necessary *conditions* for (secondary causes of) the action of the bacillus are the peculiar bodily constitution, predisposition, susceptibility and environment of the patient. Without these concomitant conditions or causes, no one would ever have tuberculosis.

Thus, in order to explain by science or accomplish by art a complex result, many laws must be considered, *but especially the law of reciprocal action.*

All changes in nature are the result of the reciprocal action (action and reaction) of bodies and forces. But here an important distinction must be made between *animate* and *inanimate* bodies and forces; between living organisms and machines.

Reciprocal action is *mediate* and *immediate.* Within the living organism, bodies and forces act *immediately,* the one upon the other, by virtue of the living fellowship of all its parts. In a machine they act *mediately*.

The motion of all parts of a machine depends, at every moment, upon the force of the external cause alone, the machine remaining constantly passive to the action of the force.

The machine cannot supply itself with oil, repair the losses it suffers from rust, friction, etc., nor reproduce itself in whole or in part. It knows no need and feels no necessity for any of these things. The living organism, on the contrary, does know and feel its need and seeks to supply it.

The living organism also receives external substances and their forces into itself, yet they are not the sole causes of its motions, but only for the nourishment of the constantly active parts.

Substances taken into the organism from without remain *passive within* the organism, while the organism toward them is *active*. Food does not pass spontaneously into the blood, nor is the blood changed spontaneously into bile or urine, but these things occur by virtue of *living,* intelligent, reciprocal causes and effects residing and taking place within the organism, according to determinate specific laws. Hence a machine is the complete opposite of an organism.

Science derives its knowledge of Life from a consideration of the facts of observation and experience in connection with the laws which express the form of their necessity, in accordance with which they occur. The facts and the laws stand together with the same objective value.

In considering the succession of two different states of the same living body, such as health and disease, the *law of causation* teaches that no internal effect can arise without an external cause, and that the effect itself may in turn become a cause of further changes.

The law of *vis inertiæ* teaches that all internal changes of bodies in nature are the results of an external cause, for without this all bodies would remain in the same state in which they were placed. The *state* of the body must be known before any change in it can be known. The cause or reason of the *state* of the body, therefore, are the *conditions* under which it can be changed by any external cause.

In Medical science and especially in therapeutics, rigid discrimination must be made between the two relations of *state* and *changes* according to these two laws (causation and *vis inertiæ*); since the action of the curative agents introduced into the body as external causes, for the purpose of changing a state of disease into a state of health, can only be determined by paying due regard to the conditions of age, sex, constitution, predisposition, etc., as manifested by symptoms or phenomena.

Regard must always be had for the differences which exist between that which is constant and unchangeable in the life of the organism and that which is changeable. The constant and unchangeable are *the laws of its specific form,* as shown in cells, connective tissue, etc. Forms are transmitted by parents. The *changeable* are the chemical and physical properties of these constituents of the organism, which are derived from the external world, and the functioning of the organism itself. Pathological form elements *must be like* the physiological, since the organism can form nothing within itself against its own unchangeable laws. According to the law of specification, every change of form or function in organism is accompanied by a corresponding changed combination of matter. Hence, when we observe any physical phenomena undergoing a change in the organism we know that chemico-vital changes are going on at the same time.

Two things thus constitute disease:—first, the *qualities of the organism,* which constitute the conditions for the disease; second, the *external causes of the disease.*

Forms of disease also obey a fixed law of constancy. Entire groups of disease, chronic and acute, and externally the most various, arise from the same morbid cause and form a unit in their *succession,* although one form occurs in childhood, another in youth and still another in advanced years. Syphilis and tuberculosis are striking examples.

Instead of seeking the cause and character of a presenting form of disease only in that which is immediate and near at hand, we should seek the more remote causes which have manifested themselves in the sequence of disorders and diseases which have preceded the present form. Upon the adoption of this principle depends the power of prevision and progress, as well as an efficient prophylaxis and therapeutics.

All functioning of the living organism depends upon a constant reciprocal action between the different constituents of the body within itself, and of the organism as a whole with its environment, the external world and its constituents.

According to the laws of causation and *vis inertiæ*, every part of the whole is at the same time active and passive, or in a state of approximate equilibrium of motion or rest. Disease, strictly speaking, is neither an action nor a reaction, but only a new or changed state of the organism caused by the interaction of an external cause with the internal constituents of the organism, resulting in a new form of the whole of a reciprocal action in which cause and effect are ever conjoined.

Physically speaking, forces are properties of substances, or bodies. They may be divided into *changeable* and *unchangeable* forces. Only those properties which are specific of bodies under all circumstances, which are necessary and constant, which isolate them perfectly from all other bodies and give each its individuality, can properly be called forces. Such, for example, are the specific gravity of each separate body; the property of a body which determines the constant equivalents of its combination with hydrogen or oxygen, or the specific individual qualities of organic forms.

Any change in bodies produced by an external cause takes place only within their changeable forces or properties, as in their volume, density, color, or manner of chemical combination.

The basic or unchangeable forces of matter which are the properties of its masses, are divided into forces of *repulsion* or *attraction*. Both may operate at a distance or by contact. Since every action in nature is a reciprocal action between bodies, such a basic force does not belong to the body alone, but belongs to it *in the ratio of its relations to other bodies*. Here we find that the like repel and the unlike attract each other.

Thus, every whole exists under the conditions of the combinations of its parts; the combination of its parts creates a dependence of the parts upon each other, and upon the specific form of the whole; and the whole exists in reciprocal relations with other forms in the external world.

Hence, in the organic world, there are no simple bodies, but only the simple, primary substance (the incorporeal life substance itself), of which, in combination with the chemical elements, all living organized bodies are formed. Even living cells are not simple, since physically they are composed of chemical elements, the fundamental forces of which differ according to their form and composition and their reciprocal relation with the life force of the organism.

Within the cells, among their constituent chemical elements, exist the basic forces of attraction and repulsion, acting reciprocally with the inherent life force of the organism, derived from the incorporeal life substance itself.

Physical science has come to regard all matter as a "condensation" of the universal, intangible, interatomic ether, which is thus acknowledged to be a fundamental substance. But physical science cannot account for *life* and *mind* or *intelligence* without acknowledging that life and mind are also substantial entities, having their existence in the being and existence of the one ineffable, omnipotent, omniscient and omnipresent Supreme Being.

Relations of Science and Art.—Art and science are inseparably bound together. Every art has its foundation in science, and every science finds its expression in art.

Consciously or unconsciously the artist or the craftsman at work is applying principles and laws, formulated and systematized knowledge of which constitutes science.

Exceptionally an artist, by virtue of inherent capacity and genius, may not be aware that he is applying scientific principles in his work. The "Art Instinct," when powerful, may express itself spontaneously and naturally by force of an internal feeling or native impulse, grasping principles intuitively and subconsciously and developing its own methods of technique through individual experience. But such endowment is rare, and even the greatest natural genius does not reach his highest development until he has awakened to the existence of theories, laws and principles and viewed his work consciously from the scientific standpoint.

When an artist reaches that point of development, philosophy begins to interest him. His eyes are opened and his vision is clear. He now wants things explained. Thenceforth, his field is broadened and his power of expression increases in proportion to his determinate development in that direction.

The scientist on the contrary never, or very rarely, proceeds by instinct. His eyes are open from the beginning. He knows exactly what he wants to do. He works deliberately by established rules and methods, based upon principles deduced from ascertained facts. Reason and logic, rather than feeling and emotion, are his guides from first to last. Not that the scientist may and does not have his moments of inspiration and high emotion as his imagination leaps forward into new fields opened up before him, or some new discovery rewards his studies, investigations and researches; for he certainly does have such moments and the greater the man, the more frequently does he experience them. When the artist becomes a scientist and the scientist becomes an artist they meet on the mountain tops of human experience and share alike in the joys of conscious creation.

Homœopathy is both an art and a science. The successful homœopathician must be both an artist and a scientist. His work must be both artistic and scientific. Theory and practice must go hand in hand. Technique must be governed by definite principles. Performance must be consistent with profession.

Some knowledge of the principles which are common to all sciences and arts is essential to a correct understanding of the special art and science with which we are concerned as homœopathicians. Study of the relation of homœopathy to other arts and sciences has been neglected and the standards as well as the morale of the profession have been lowered in consequence.

Homœopathy has been regarded too much as a thing apart; a wanderer without friends or relations; a sort of medical Topsy: "Never had no parents—jes' growed." The fact is that homœopathy was the logical and legitimate offspring of the Inductive Philosophy and Method of Aristotle and Lord Bacon. It is the highest development of modern therapeutic science and as such stands intimately related to the sciences of Logic, Mathematics, Physics, Chemistry, Biology, Psychology and other sciences. The broader and more accurate the knowledge of these relations, the higher will be the respect for and the warmer the enthusiasm in the practice of the Hahnemannian Art.

Fundamental conceptions of matter and motion; energy and force; spirit and life; mind and body; health and disease; cure and recovery and their relations to each other which are embodied in the Organon of Hahnemann and which I shall endeavor to interpret in the light of modern science and philosophy, are not only the profoundest subjects of human thought, but they are an integral part of homœopathy.

Realization of this fact should arouse interest. It stimulates the kind of thought and study which develop the scientific spirit. It is the most powerful factor in the creation of that high *morale* which is so essential to the progress and perpetuation of the science of therapeutic medication. The highest loyalty to principles, consistency in practice and perfection of methods can be attained in no other way.

A carpenter who is content to know his steel square only as a tool by which he can measure or draw a straight line across a board and tell whether the angles of a frame are true, will never become anything more than a mere day laborer. But arouse his interest in the mysterious lines and figures on that wonderful instrument; induct him into the mathematics of the square; teach him its higher uses and the possibilities of his development and progress are almost unlimited.

So the physician who knows only a little rudimentary materia medica and therapeutics in addition to his medical-college knowledge of general medicine, and is content with that knowledge, will never be anything but a routinist and a medical misfit.

Homœopathy a Science.—Homœopathy, or homœotherapy, is the department of science in general medicine which has for its principal objects the observation and study of the action of remedial agents in health and disease, and the treatment and cure of disease by medication, according to a fixed law or general principle.

Homœopathy was founded and developed into a scientific

GENERAL INTERPRETATIONS

system by Samuel Hahnemann (1755-1843) under the principles of the Inductive Method of Science as developed by Lord Bacon. Its practice is governed by the principle of Symptom-Similarity, which is the application in medicine of the universal principle of Mutual Action formulated by Sir Isaac Newton in his Third Law of Motion: "Action and reaction are equal and opposite."

Homœopathy, as a science, rests fundamentally upon four general principles: Similarity, Contrariety, Proportionality and Infinitesimality, reducible to the universal principle of Homœosis, or Universal Assimilation. (Fincke.)

"Science is Knowledge reduced to law and embodied in system." "Knowledge of a single fact, not known as related to any other, or of many facts, not known as having any mutual relations or as comprehended under any general law, does not reach the meaning of science."

"A science in its development is 1. A collection of exactly observed facts; 2. A correlation or generalization of these facts, forming a system; 3. A formulation of these generalizations as laws; 4. It proceeds to some principle or force accounting for these laws; hence, exact knowledge of proximate causes." (Condensed from The Standard Dictionary.)

Law, in the broadest sense, is the observed order or relation of the facts. It is not required that the cause of the order or relation be known. As mathematicians and astronomers, accustomed to deal with the highest order of facts, are content to accept the law of gravitation without explanation of the cause, so physicians, if there be a law of cure, may accept it without explanation of its cause. But the tendency of modern physical science is toward the more complete generalization, its goal being the discovery of a universal principle which shall connect all physical phenomena.

Specifically, in the scientific sense, a law is the connecting link between two series of phenomena, showing their relation to each other.

"There are two tests of the validity of any law that is claimed to be a natural law, or law of nature.

1. That it is capable of connecting and explaining two series of natural phenomena.

2. That it is in harmony with other known laws.

In optics, for example, we have the phenomena or properties of luminous bodies, and the phenomena of light receiving bodies. These two series of phenomena are connected and explained by the law of the diffusion of light.

In physics the phenomena of the sun, as regards density and volume, are related to the phenomena of the earth by the law of attraction or gravitation.

In chemistry the properties of potassium are related to the properties of sulphuric acid by the law of chemical affinity and definite proportions, in the formation of a new compound, potassium sulphate." (Abstracted from Dunham, Science of Therapeutics.)

So in Homœotherapy, we have the phenomena of drugs related to the phenomena of diseases by the law of mutual action, under the principles of similarity, contrariety, proportionality and infinitesimality; reducible again to the principle of Universal Assimilation or Homœosis.

"Therapeutics is that department of medical science that relates to the treatment of disease and the action of remedial agents on the human organism, both in health and disease." (Standard Dictionary.)

Since it conforms to every requirement of these general, authoritative definitions of Science, homœopathy has been defined as The Science of Therapeutics. No other method or system of medical treatment conforms or even claims to conform to all of these fundamental requirements.

But while it can easily be shown that the curative action of any agent whatsoever used in the treatment of disease, mental or physical, conforms to the fundamental principle of Mutual Action, in the narrower or more practical sense homœopathy must be defined as *the science of therapeutic medication,* since it commonly uses medicines or drugs alone to effect its purposes.

Homœopathy is not, strictly speaking, "a system of medicine" as it is often inaccurately called, using the word medicine in its broad general sense. General medicine is made up of a number of distinct sciences, including General Therapeutics, which covers all the therapeutic resources known to man. It makes use of many agencies besides medication for the alleviation of human ills.

Homœopathy, therefore, is a department of general medicine, like anatomy, physiology and pathology.

Homœopathy an Experimental Science.—Like chemistry or physics, homœopathy is established under the principles of the inductive method in science. Considered as a science, it consists of two series of phenomena, independently observed, collected and studied, connected by an underlying law or principle of nature. Its elements are: 1, The phenomena of disease; 2, the phenomena produced by drugs when administered to healthy persons; and 3, the general law of mutual action, otherwise known as Newton's Third Law of Motion and as the Law of Similars, which connects the two series of phenomena. The phenomena of disease constitute its pathology, the experimentally derived phenomena of drugs, its materia medica and the application of its materia medica under the law its therapeutics.

Experimentally, in the construction of homœopathic materia medica, medicines were administered singly, in various doses, to healthy human beings for the purpose of eliciting, observing, recording and comparing their effects. Comparison shows that the symptoms thus produced by drugs are similar to the symptoms of disease. Any symptom or group of symptoms of disease may be duplicated from the materia medica record of drug symptoms.

Experimentally also it has been proven that under certain conditions, to be stated hereafter, medicines cure diseases by virtue of their similarity of symptoms; that is, medicines cure, or remove in the sick, symptoms similar to those which they have the power of producing in the healthy. From this fact of experience was deduced the law of cure and medication, known as the "law of similars," which is found on examination to be a statement in other words of the general Law of Mutual Action, variously termed the law of equivalence, the law of action and reaction, the law of balance or equilibrium, the law of polarity, the law of compensation and Newton's third law of motion.

Homœopathy an Art.—Homœopathy works in perfect harmony with all necessary rational, non-medicinal and mechanical therapeutic agents. Surgery, obstetrics, hygiene, dietetics, sanitary science, chemistry (so far as it is applied in the preparation of medicines and in ejecting and antidoting poisons) and psycho-therapy all find in homœopathy their congenial and most powerful ally.

Homœopathy is opposed in its constitution and principles to all forms of treatment by direct or physiological medication, and to physio-chemical treatment or treatment based upon chemical theories.

Homœopathy is opposed to the use, under ordinary conditions, of drugs in physiological doses for mere palliative purposes, since its primary object is always the cure or obliteration of disease and complete restoration of health.

Homœopathy is opposed to the *methods* of vaccine and serum therapy, although it is claimed by many that these methods are based upon the homœopathic principle. It grants that this may be true so far as the underlying principle is concerned, but opposes *the method of applying the principle* as being a violation of sound, natural principles of medication and productive of serious injury to the living organism.

It has been proven experimentally and clinically that such methods are unnecessary, and that the results claimed by their advocates can be attained more safely, more rapidly and more thoroughly by the administration of the homœopathically indicated medicines in sub-physiological doses, through the natural channels of the body, than by introducing it forcibly by means of the hypodermic needle or in any other way.

Homœopathy is opposed to so-called "pathological prescribing" and to "group treatment" of diseases, by which individual peculiarities are ignored and patients are grouped or classed according to their gross, pathological organic lesions and treated alike. Homœopathy deals with the individual, not the class. It treats *the patient,* not a fictitious entity called the disease. Its prescription or selection of medicines is based solely upon individual similarity of symptoms, drug symptoms to disease symptoms, determined by actual comparison in each case.

Homœopathy is opposed to all forms of external, local or topical drug treatment of the external, secondary symptoms of disease, except in surgical cases. It directs its curative agents through the natural channels of the body to the physiological centers of vital action and reaction, which govern all functional activities in the living organism in disease as well as in health.

Homœopathy is opposed to polypharmacy. It depends for all its results upon the dynamical action of single, pure, potentiated medicines, prepared by a special mathematico-mechanical process and administered in minimum doses.

In practice, homœopathy bases the selection of the curative remedy upon the totality of the symptoms of the individual patient, including a consideration of the ascertainable causes of the disease. For the homœopathic prescriber this constitutes the disease. Speculation as to the inner, essential nature or workings of the drug or the disease does not enter into the process of selecting the remedy. The prescription is not based upon the pathological diagnosis, or the name of the disease, but solely upon the likeness of the symptoms of the patient to the symptoms of some tested drug, determined by actual comparison.

As the experimental work in constructing the homœopathic materia medica has been conducted with single medicines, and as each medicine has its own definite and peculiar kind and sphere of action, scientific accuracy, as well as the law of similars, requires that the treatment of patients be conducted in the same manner. Medicines are never mixed or compounded in homœopathic practice but are given singly.

It has been proven experimentally that the sick organism is peculiarly and even painfully sensitive to the action of the single, similar medicine, and that curative effects are only obtained by sub-physiological doses. Physiological doses, instead of removing the symptoms of the disease, produce by their direct pathogenetic action the characteristic symptom of the drug. If the drug be not a similar the condition of the patient is complicated by the addition of symptoms having no relation to the disease and no cure results. If the drug be a similar the violent reaction of the organism to the unnecessarily large dose increases suffering, exhausts the patient and prolongs his disease, even if he eventually recovers.

These facts led, first, to the progressive reduction of the size of the dose to the smallest effectual curative quantity, and eventually to the discovery and formulation of *the law of potentiation and the infinitesimal dose,* which is one of the corollaries of the law of similars and a fundamental principle of homœopathy.

The working principles of homœopathy, therefore, may be briefly stated as follows:

1. The totality of the symptoms of the patient is the basis of medical treatment.

2. The use of single medicines, the symptoms and sphere of action of which have been predetermined by pure, controlled experiments upon healthy persons.

3. The principle of symptom-similarity as the guide to the choice of the remedy.

4. The minimum dose capable of producing a dynamic or functional reaction. *Similia Similibus Curentur; Simplex. Simile Minimum.*

CHAPTER III

Schools of Philosophy

It will be well to take a glance at the various schools of philosophy in order to be able to understand his point of view and identify the fundamental ideas and concepts out of which Hahnemann developed his system.

The various schools of philosophy may be broadly classified as materialistic, idealistic and substantialistic.

Materialism.—"The doctrine that the facts of experience are all to be explained by reference to the reality, activities and laws of physical or material substance. In psychology this doctrine denies the reality of the soul as psychical being; in cosmology, it denies the need of assuming the being of God as Absolute Spirit or of any other spiritual ground or first principle; opposed to spiritualism. Materialistic theories have varied from the first, but the most widely accepted form regards all species of sentiment and mental life as *products of organism*, and the universe itself as resolvable into terms of physical elements and their motions." (Standard Dictionary.)

Here we should consider for a moment the meaning of the words "reality" and "substance." The "dyed in the wool" materialist regards nothing as real and substantial which has not *tangibility*. He reduces everything to the terms of physical matter, which is for him the only reality. If he uses the words, energy, power, force, motion, principle, law, mind, life or thought, which represent intangible things, it is to regard them merely as attributes, conditions or products of matter. For him the things represented are neither real or substantial. They exist, as it were, only in the imagination. Because they are not tangible they are not real. Not being real, according to his way of looking at things, they are not substantial and, therefore, are not worthy of consideration. The fact that he is compelled to act as if they were real makes no difference in his mental attitude. He refuses to admit their existence as anything but properties of matter.

The unfortunate thing about this philosophy is that it seems to induce and foster a peculiarly irritating, skeptical, antagonistic and unscientific frame of mind toward many things which others feel and know in their inmost consciousness to be very real indeed—ideas which are the source and substance of their deepest convictions, highest aspirations and most illuminating conceptions. This attitude may and often does become offensive in the extreme, largely because it is so one-sided, and those who hold it refuse so obstinately to "call things by their right names." To the broader and more philosophic mind the intangible, invisible energy, power, principle, law or intelligence is as real and as substantial as the material things which it creates and controls and should be so denominated in all frankness and sincerity.

Idealism.—"That system of reflective thinking which would interpret and explain the whole universe, things and minds and their relations, as the realization of a system of ideas. It takes various forms as determined by the view of what the idea or the ideal is, and of how we become aware of it." (*Vide*.)

Substantialism.—"The doctrine that substantial existences or real beings are the sources or underlying ground of all phenomena, mental and material; especially the doctrine which denies that the conception of material substance can be resolved into mere centers of force." (*Vide*.)

The fundamental idea of Substantialism is ancient, but the systematic development and application of it is modern.

"The predominant thought of substantialism is that all things in Nature which exist or can form the basis of a concept are really substantial entities, whether they are the so-called principles or forces of nature or the atoms of corporeal bodies, even extending to the life and mental powers of every sentient organism, from the highest to the lowest." (Hall.)

It holds, for example, that the "wave theory" of sound is a fallacy in science. Hall experimentally established the fact that;—"Sound consists of corpuscular emissions and is therefore a substantial entity, as much so as air or odor." He argues;—"If sound can be proved to be a substance there cannot be the shadow of a scientific objection raised against the substantial or entitative nature of life and the mental powers." From this point of view, mind is as real in its existence as is the physical brain, which is regarded as the tangible manifestation of the form and substance of its invisible counterpart.

"If mind is the result of the motion of the molecules of the brain, of what does that result consist? If the motion of the molecules is the all of mind, then the mind is nothing, a nonentity, since motion itself is a nonentity." (Hall.)

From nothing, nothing comes. Every effect proceeds from a cause. Effects follow causes in unbroken succession.

No substantial effect can be produced upon any subject without an absolute substance of some kind connecting the cause with the effect.

Gravity, or that which produces gravitation, is a substance, since it acts upon physical objects at a distance and causes substantial physical effects.

Magnetism is a substance, since it passes through imporous bodies, seizes upon and moves iron.

Sound is a substance, since it is "conveyed through space by air waves." It must be something substantial or it could not be conveyed.

Light, heat and (or) electricity are (is) substantial. (They may be identical.) It is absurd to call them "modes of motion" or "vibratory phenomena." Motion is a non-entity, the mere act of a thing in changing its position in space. Motion is nothing before an object begins to move, and nothing after it has ceased to move. Modern science teaches that light and heat are motions or vibrations of *the ether.* Physical science, therefore, tacitly teaches that the ether is substantial; has measured it; has calculated its inertia-coefficient and its kinetic energy; has pronounced it to be the primary substance of which matter as well as heat, light and electricity, is composed. If science is right in this theory then light, heat and electricity are substantial emanations from their producing bodies or substances; in other words, they are each composed of ether, *varying in its rate of vibration.* But physical science (materialism) does not tell us *who* or *what* moves the ether and determines the rate of vibration. That remains for substantialism, which teaches that Life is *a substance,* having the qualities of a **real,** entitative being. By its agency alone organized, living, con-

3

scious, thinking, willing entities are created, maintained and reproduced. Hence, Life is intelligent, else it could not manifest these qualities.

Mind is a substance, since it acts to think or produce thoughts and things. Mind, therefore, has intelligence. Thought—the action of mind—may be called "a mode of motion of mind, acting upon the molecules of the brain." In the last analysis *life and mind are one and identical,* since they have identical qualities and attributes, and Mind (Syn: life, spirit) is the primary cause of motion. *Life is energy, and all energy is living energy.*

As regards living beings, including man, the substantialistic hypothesis is:—"that within every living creature there exists a vital and mental organism, the (invisible) counterpart of the physical structure, the source of all vital and physiological phenomena, originally contributed by the Creative Will (Mind—Life—Spirit) as atoms out of His own being, and which must at the dissolution of organic life return to the vital and mental fountain whence they emanated, there to mingle by reabsorption into the original source, or, as in the case of those (human) lives which have received the spiritual impress of God's image, live forever with the self-conscious ego inherited through their higher organism." (Hall.)

Hahnemann's Position.—Hahnemann has heretofore been assigned to the Idealists. In an attempt to be more definite he has been called a "Vitalist," referring to the prominence given in The Organon to the doctrine of life and vital force.

In advance of the appearance of substantialism as a formulated philosophy and a name, this was perhaps the best that could be done in the attempt to classify Hahnemann philosophically. But since a definite philosophy has been formulated there can be no question that he is properly classified as a substantialist. His position and statements in regard to the Deity; to life, mind, vital force, matter, potentization (or dynamization), infinitesimals, and the emphasis he lays upon the substantial character of these (to him) great realities do not fully agree with any other classification. Hahnemann frankly and reverently recognizes The Supreme Being, as indeed every scientific man must do who thinks logically straight through to the end. Otherwise all thought ends in negation.

Hahnemann's constant appeal to experience, to facts of observation and experiment, and to the necessity in medicine of avoiding speculation of all kinds, establishes the practical, well-balanced character of his mind. He refused to speculate about the essential nature of things. He observed and accepted the facts of existence as he saw them. To him, spirit and matter, force and motion, mind and body, health and disease, in all their mutations and modifications, *co-exist* as facts of observation, consciousness and experience. It was for him to use them in a logical and practical manner. He was not a materialist who denied the deific origin and existence of spiritual substances or agents, and maintained that spiritual or mental phenomena are the result of some peculiar organization of matter. Neither was he an idealist in the extreme sense of one who believed, with Bishop Berkeley (and Mrs. Eddy) that all which exists is spirit, and that which is called matter, or the external world, is either a succession of notions impressed on the mind by Deity, an illusion or "error," or else the mere edict of the mind itself as taught by Fichte.

The Inductive Philosophy of Lord Bacon.—Familiarity with the works and doctrines of the philosophers is shown in Hahnemann's writings; but he seems to have been most influenced by the inductive philosophy of Lord Bacon. He never mentioned nor quoted Bacon in his writings, but few finer examples of the application of Bacon's principle to the study of natural phenomena can be found than that of Hahnemann in his development of Homœopathy.

Bacon had set himself particularly to the task of a complete investigation and reformation of physical science; but his plan embraced the whole realm of philosophy, and his principle was applicable to mental and moral, no less than physical science. That principle was Logical Induction, upon which was based the inductive method of observation and experience. This is the only valid basis of conclusions and the accepted ground of modern science.

"His (Bacon's) merit as a philosopher lies chiefly in having called back the human mind from the wrong direction in which it had so long been seeking knowledge, and setting it on a new path of investigation," says one writer.

"When Bacon had analyzed the philosophy of the ancients, he

found it speculative. The great highways of life had been deserted. Nature, spread out to the intelligence of man, . . . had scarcely been consulted by the ancient philosophers. They had looked within and not without. They had sought to rear systems on the uncertain foundations of human hypothesis and speculation instead of resting them on the immutable laws of Providence as manifested in the material world. Bacon broke the bars of this mental prison-house:—bade the mind go free and investigate nature." (Davies, Logic of Mathematics.)

Bacon's fame rests chiefly on his *"Novum Organum,"* the second part of his *"Instauratio Magna."* "The object of this was to furnish the world a better mode of investigation of truth; that is, a better logic than the so-called Aristotelian or syllogistic method; a logic of which the aim should be not to supply arguments for controversy, but to investigate nature, and by observation and the complete induction of particulars arrive at truth."

It is significant that Hahnemann in selecting a name for his own *Magnum Opus* chose the very word, "Organon," used by Bacon, and before him by Aristotle, whose philosophical method, misrepresented and misapplied by the schoolmen of the middle ages, Bacon restored to its true place with improvements of his own.

State of Medicine in Hahnemann's Time.—The situation confronting Hahnemann in the medical world was similar in many respects to that in the world of physical science which confronted Bacon. Medical theory trod upon the heels of theory as they rapidly passed across the historical field of vision, each one contradicting the other, and all alike the product of imagination and speculation. All were engaged in attempting to find a basis for the treatment of disease in speculations about the interior states, the invisible, internal changes in the organs of the body and the unknowable primary causes of disease.

Ideas which now seem absurd were then matters of the most serious moment, and in their practical working out often became tragical. Blood-letting, the outgrowth of one of these false theories, affords a good example. The celebrated Bouvard, physician to Louis XIII, ordered his royal patient forty-seven bleedings, two hundred and fifteen emetics or purgatives, and three hundred and twelve clysters during the period of one year! During the extremes to which the so-called "physiological medicine" was carried more than six million leeches were used, and more than two hundred thousand pounds of blood was spilled in the hospitals of Paris in one year. The mortality was appalling.

In Hahnemann's time (1799) the death of our own George Washington was undoubtedly caused by the repeated bloodletting to which he was subjected. He was almost completely exsanguinated.

Medicine was in a state of chaos. Hahnemann faced the problem of creating a new science and art of therapeutics which should be constructed on the basis of facts of observation and experience, according to certain principles which he had laid down for his guidance.

Applying the inductive method which he had evidently learned from Bacon and Aristotle, the first thing Hahnemann did was to take a broad view of the whole field of medicine, shake himself clear of any lingering remnant of bias or prejudice which may have been in his mind as a result of his association with the medical men and ideas of his age, and ask himself a few simple, pointed questions.

"What is the real mission of the physician?" "Of what use is the medical profession?" "Has it any real excuse to offer for its existence?" "Surely not," he says, "if it spends its time and effort in concocting so-called systems out of empty vagaries and hypotheses concerning the inner obscure nature of the process of life; or the origin of disease; nor in the innumerable attempts at explaining the phenomena of diseases or their proximate causes, ever hidden from their scrutiny, which they clothe in unintelligible words; or as a mass of abstract phrases intended for the astonishment of the ignorant, while suffering humanity was sighing for help. We have had more than enough of such learned absurdities called theoretical medicine, having its own professorships, and it is high time for those who call themselves physicians to cease deluding poor humanity by idle words, and to begin to act, that is, to help and to heal."

"The physician's highest and only calling is to restore health to the sick, which is called Healing."

"Rational Medicine."—Scientific medicine must conform to at least three requirements: 1. It must be based on facts. 2. It must be rational, that is, logical. 3. It must be demonstrably true.

It is not enough for medicine to be simply "rational." When people believed that epidemics were sent by offended deities it was "rational" that their children should be offered as propitiatory sacrifices. If one believes that disease is merely an "error of mortal mind" it will be "rational" to adopt the methods of Mrs. Eddy. So-called "rational medicine," since the days of Hippocrates (whose "four humors," "humoral diseases" and "humoral remedies" still exist, masquerading under the thinly-disguised term "serum therapy"), has always been "rational," but too often neither logical, based on facts, nor demonstrably true.

What a confession of ignorance of the healing art and of blind worship of false gods is contained in the following paragraphs from a recent editorial in a prominent medical journal:

"No record in history equals the death roll of the World War and the accompanying pandemic of influenza. In these two giant convulsions *man was helpless.*

"In the struggle against influenza medicine and science could salvage only a few. If we should experience a recurrence of the epidemic, either mild or severe, are we prepared to meet it?"

Statistics of the epidemic referred to show a total loss under "regular" treatment of approximately a million lives in the United States, with a mortality rate of about thirty per cent!

A hecatomb indeed on the altars of modern "rational medicine," the frightfulness of which is brought home to us by the fact that in fifty thousand cases reported by homœopathic physicians the mortality was only about one per cent!

Hahnemann's Working Principles.—It will be profitable to glance at some general principles which Hahnemann laid down for his guidance in his great work of creating a new science and art of therapeutics. These are to be found succinctly stated in the preface to the second edition of the Organon.

He there broadly defines medicine as "a pure science of experience, like physics and chemistry."

He declares: "Medicine can and must rest on clear facts and sensible phenomena, for all the subjects it has to deal with are clearly cognizable by the senses through experience. Knowledge of the disease to be treated, knowledge of the effects of the medicine and how the ascertained effects of the medicines are to be employed for the removal of disease—all this is taught adequately by experience, and by experience alone. Its subjects can only be derived from pure experience and observations, and it dare not take a single step out of the sphere of pure, well-observed experience and experiments, if it would avoid becoming a nullity and a farce.'

He continues: "Unaided reason can know nothing of itself (*a priori*), can evolve out of itself alone no conception of the nature of things, of cause and effects; its conclusions about the actual must always be based upon sensible perceptions, facts and experiences if it would elicit truth. If in its operation it should deviate by a single step from the guidance of perception it would lose itself in the illimitable region of phantasy and of arbitrary speculation, the mother of pernicious illusion and of absolute nullity."

"Such," he says, "has hitherto been the splendid juggling of so-called theoretical medicine, in which *a priori* conceptions and speculative subtleties only showed things which could not be known, and which were of no use for the cure of disease.

"In the pure sciences of experience," he continues, "in physics, chemistry and medicine, merely speculative reason can consequently have no voice; there, when it acts alone, it degenerates into empty speculation and phantasy and produces only hazardous hypotheses which are, and by their very nature must be, self-deceptive and false."

Ameke, the historian of homœopathy, has made an illuminating comment on the last quoted paragraph. He says: "The great difference between Hahnemann and the later natural historical school is expressed by himself in one small word of three letters: —'and.' Hahnemann speaks of 'physics, chemistry *and* medicine'; they said; 'medicine is applied physics and chemistry,' and founded medicine on these two sciences." Hahnemann founded medicine, not on physics and chemistry, but on *the universal laws of Life and Motion*.

Hahnemann starts, then, with the conception of **Life as a** real or substantial entitative power or principle, having laws of its own, and refers all the phenomena of health and disease to it under two names: "The Dynamis" and "The Life Force." *This is Hahnemann's greatest discovery, and the absolute bed-rock of his system.*

The words "force" and "life force" were used inaccurately in this connection, however, making it difficult for some to form a clear conception of what life is in its philosophical relation to homœopathy. The failure to make a distinction between *power* and *force* has always caused confusion. The word "force" generally, as well as in the Organon, is loosely used to express the idea of any operating or operative power or energy; of any active agency or power tending to change the state of matter; and this is the sense in which Hahnemann often uses the word in the Organon when he speaks of the "life force" as that which acts and is acted upon in disease and cure.

Now, as a matter of fact, we do not act upon force nor upon motion. These terms express abstract ideas or concepts which stand to the concrete things or reality back of them in the relation of effects to causes.

Force and motion are merely phenomena of the power which produces them. Power is the property of any thing or substance by virtue of which it is able to produce changes in itself, or in any other thing or substance.

Motion is the result of the application of force. Force is the product of power or energy. The power inherent in a body is quite another thing from the force exerted by it or upon it.

Action (motion) takes place only in or in connection with that which has the power to react or resist, the thing itself, whether it be a stone, a machine or a living organism. The thing itself is always substantial, having a real objective existence, even if it be intangible or invisible. Strictly speaking, we do not act upon the life force, but upon life itself, the real, substantial, objective, although intangible, substance from which the living organism is evolved, of which it is composed and from which the life force proceeds.

The organism does not evolve out of nothing. "Out of nothing, nothing comes." The living organism is a development, an evolution from a microscopic cell, which is itself an organism composed of living matter and a nucleus, developed from invisible, living substance which attracts to itself, assimilates and transforms tangible elements from the material world.

Everything living comes from preceding life in an unbroken chain, the last conceivable link of which is in the one Infinite and Eternal Source of Life, the Supreme Being. Metaphysical science recognizes this conception under the term of "The Cosmic Life."

In thinking upon this subject it is necessary, in order to avoid confusion, to keep clearly in mind the distinction between the Thing Itself and its action. There can be no action without something to act; no phenomena without the being of which the phenomena are an expression; no force without the power which exerts the force; no thought without a thinker. The words, action, phenomena, force, thought, stand for abstract ideas, separated from the real, substantial things or causes which lie back of them, for purposes of thought.

We do not see motion; we see a body change its position in space, as when one picks up a book from one side of the desk and places it on the other side. We do not see force; we see the effects of force upon a body in changing its position in space. We do not see life; we see only its manifestation in organism. But knowing intuitively and by experience that there can be no effect without a cause, no motion without force, and no force without something or somebody to exercise power, we assume the existence of that power, person or thing as a primitive fact and name it, although we cannot see the power, person or thing with the physical eye, even with the aid of an ultra microscope. We see the primary substance, power, person or thing with the mental eye and are satisfied.

To refuse to see and acknowledge the substance, principle, power or person behind the force, and to confine thinking within the limits of matter, phenomena and force is to kill the highest aspirations of the soul, stultify the intellect and land the thinker in the morass of materialism. A certain class of thinkers, especially in physical science, plume themselves upon their rigid limitation of thought within the bounds of physical phenomena. They deny not only the validity of any attempt to see what lies beyond phenomena, but the reality and substantial existence of anything lying beyond that arbitrary boundary. Metaphysics is their pet aversion. Such men invariably entangle themselves in a maze of contradictions and absurdities and mislead their followers. They juggle with words, invert the terms of logical propositions, formulate "circular syllogisms" and make causes follow effects.

Metaphysical thought and inquiry are quite as legitimate and valid, and quite as capable of being conducted logically and scientifically, as physical research. There is a valid and scientific metaphysics as well as physics.

George Henry Lewes says: "It is experience—our own or that of others—on which we rest. We are not at liberty to invent experience, nor to infer anything contrary to it, only to extend it analogically. Speculation to be valid must be simply the extension of experience by the analogies of experiences. * * * It is possible to move securely in the ground of speculation so long as we carefully pick our way, and consider each position insecure till what was merely probable becomes proven."

Hahnemann at first apparently had the distinction between power and force pretty clearly in mind in his use, in the Organon, of the two terms: "Dynamis," the life power, the substance, the thing itself, objectively considered; and "Life-Force," the action of the power; but he failed to maintain the distinction uniformly in his subsequent use of the words. All doubt as to Hahnemann's ultimate position is removed and the subject is placed beyond controversy, so far as he is concerned, however, by the final sixth revised edition of the Organon which is at last accessible to the profession. In this edition Hahnemann invariably uses the term, *Vital Principle* instead of Vital Force, even speaking in one place of *"the vital force of the Vital Principle,"* thus making it clear that he held firmly to the substantialistic view of life—that is, that Life is a substantial, objective entity; a primary, originating power or principle, and not a mere condition, or "mode of motion."

From this conception arises the dynamical theory of disease upon which is based the Hahnemannian pathology, viz.:—*that disease is always primarily a dynamical (or functional) disturbance of the vital principle*. Upon this is reared the entire edifice of therapeutic medication, governed by the law of *similia* as a selective principle.

Life then is not primarily a phenomenon. It is the cause of phenomena. Life is not, strictly speaking, a force; it is a substance, a power or principle which acts to exert or cause force. Life is a substantial, self-existent, self-acting entity, not a mere abstraction. Life is not a product; it is the producer, whether it be of matter or motion. In brief, Life is intelligent, incorporeal vital substance—the original "simple substance" of the ancients.

Life, in a dynamical sense, is *energy*—the universal principle and cause of vital action and reaction, organization, growth, self-preservation and reproduction, inherent in all living things.

Life, therefore, is included under the general principle of science, which declares that "all force is persistent and indestructible;" *and this is the scientific statement of the doctrine of Immortality.*

Energy must exist before work can be done. Hence, life and mind logically and necessarily precede organization, and thus must be not only the cause but the controlling power of organization. Life built the body and life preserves it, as long as it is needed for the purpose of "our indwelling rational spirit," as Hahnemann calls it.

All schools of modern philosophy now agree that "life can come only from previous life." As a scientific doctrine the theory of "spontaneous generation," after centuries of stubbornly contested existence, has been abandoned by all except a very few stubborn persons of the materialistic school who still cling to the ancient fallacy, unaware that the ground has been cut from under them and that they have been left, like Mahomet's coffin, suspended in midair.

Step by step, with many long periods of inactivity and sometimes of retrogression, the search for the origin of life has gone on. Repeatedly, when brought up against the logical necessity of taking the final step and acknowledging the One Infinite and Eternal Source of Life, the searchers have stubbornly turned back and begun over again, only to return to the same inescapable point.

Chemist, physicist and biologist alike, each in his own special path, pursues it to the end, and there finds himself standing with his fellows on the brink of the great mystery which can only be solved by admitting the existence of The Supreme Being.

The chemist, guided by the law of chemical affinity and molecular attraction, reaches the sphere of Universal Attraction. He stops and turns away. The biologist, tracing life back through organism to the cell, and still further back to the formless bit of protoplasm lying, as it were, on the shore of the infinite ocean of his life, also halts and turns away rather than spread the sails of his little bark and sail by faith, if he must, into the haven which is in plain view if he will but open his eyes and look. The physicist analyses matter, divides and subdivides it until it disappears in the hypothetical, inanimate, unintelligent ether of space which he conceives to be the source both of matter and force, and there he also halts. Each is unsatisfied and must ever remain so until, like Hahnemann, he yields to that innermost urge of the soul which demands of every man that he take the final step and acknowledge the Infinite Life and Mind of the Universe, the source and substance of all power, the Father Eternal, to whom he owes spiritual allegiance.

CHAPTER IV

The Scope of Homœopathy

Accuracy and efficiency in homœopathic therapeutics is only possible to those who have a clearly defined idea of the field in which the principle of *Similia* is operative.

The scope of homœopathy is a subject which has received too little consideration by teachers and practitioners alike. Hazy and confused ideas prevail. As a result we find on the one hand a few sincere but misguided enthusiasts attempting the impossible and bringing ridicule upon themselves, and on the other hand, the great majority, ignorant of the higher possibilities, missing their opportunities and bringing discredit upon themselves and their art by resorting to unhomœopathic measures in cases which could readily be cured by homœopathic remedies. One believes too much, the other too little. Neither one knows why he succeeds in one case and fails in another.

Haphazard cures do not justify boasting. The art of pharmaco-therapeutics in general, and of homœopathy in particular, is not advanced by such work. What we need is clean-cut, scientific work; work capable of being rationally explained and verified; results attained by the intelligent application of a definite principle and a perfected technic in a sharply delimited field.

The therapeutic principle is known; the technic of prescribing has been developed; a large number of remedies have been prepared; but the field of action has not been clearly defined.

In this respect we are like an army which is wasting much good ammunition trying to search out a hidden enemy of whose exact location it is ignorant.

A philosophical aëroplane, sent into the upper regions of the air, may be able to locate the enemy exactly and enable us to train our guns directly upon him.

Homœopathy as a therapeutic method is concerned primarily only with the *morbid vital processes in the living organism, which are perceptibly represented by the symptoms, irrespective of what caused them.*

In defining the scope of homœopathy it is necessary first to discriminate between disease *per se,* as a morbid vital process and the material results or products in which the morbid process ultimates. With the latter, homœopathy primarily has nothing to do. It is concerned only with disease *per se,* in its primary, functional or dynamical aspect.

Disease *per se,* Hahnemann says, is "nothing more than an alteration in the state of health of a healthy individual," caused by the dynamic action of external, inimical forces *upon the life principle of the living organism,* making itself known only by perceptible signs and symptoms, the totality of which *represents* and for all practical purposes constitutes the disease.

It becomes necessary, therefore, in homœopathic prescribing to carefully separate the primary, functional symptoms which represent the morbid process itself, from the secondary symptoms which represent the pathological end-products of the disease.

The gross, tangible lesions and products in which disease ultimates are not the primary object of the homœopathic prescription. We do not prescribe for the tumor which affects the patient, nor are we guided by the secondary symptoms which arise from the mere physical presence of the tumor: We prescribe for *the patient*—selecting and being guided by the symptoms which represent the morbid, vital process which preceded, accompanied and ultimated in the development of the tumor.

If there is doubt as to which symptoms are primary and which are secondary the history will decide. In the evolution of disease in the living organism, functional changes precede organic or structural changes. *"Function creates the organ,"* is a maxim in biological and morphological science, from which it follows that *function reveals the condition of the organ.*

The order in which the symptoms of a case appear, therefore, enables us to determine which are primary and which secondary, as well as to ascribe reflex symptoms to their source and correctly localize the disease.

For the homœopathic prescriber the totality of the functional symptoms of the patient is the disease, in the sense that such symptoms constitute the only perceptible form of the disease and are the only rational basis of curative treatment. Symptoms are the outwardly perceptible signs or phenomena of internal morbid changes in the state of the previously healthy organism, and are our only means of knowing what disease is. They represent a change from a state of order to a state of disorder. When the symptoms are removed the disease ceases to exist.

These phenomena result from and represent the action upon the living organism of some external agent or influence inimical to life. With the morbific agents themselves homœopathy primarily has no more to do than it has with the tangible products or ultimates of disease. It is taken for granted that the physician, acting in another capacity than that of a prescriber of homœopathic medicine, will remove the causes of the disease and the obstacles to cure as far as possible before he addresses himself to the task of selecting and administering the remedy which is homœopathic to the symptoms of the case, by which the cure is to be performed.

In thus focusing attention upon the individual and purely functional side of disease, upon disease *per se,* the sphere of homœopathy may be clearly perceived.

From this point of view, the most significant and general feature to be observed about the phenomena or disease is the fact of motion, action, change; change of states, forms and positions; change resulting from the application of morbific force in the living organism; change from a state of health to a state of disease; and the reverse; change of symptoms and their groupings; change of order to disorder; change of form of diseased structures; change of function; change of molecular combination and arrangement; everywhere motion, change and transformation so long as life lasts. In one word, we find ourselves in the realm of *pure dynamics.* This is the true and only sphere of homœopathy, *the sphere of vital dynamics.* In fact, homœopathy might well be defined as the Science of Vital Dynamics. Its field is the field of disordered vital phenomena and functional changes in the individual patient, irrespective of the name of the disease, or of its cause. Its object is the restoration of order and harmony in vital functioning in the individual patient. Its laws are the laws of motion operating in the vital realm, which govern all vital action. Its fundamental principle is the universal principle of Mutual Action. "Action and Reaction are Equal and Opposite."

"The unprejudiced observer," says Hahnemann, "well aware of the futility of transcendental speculation which can receive no confirmation from experience—be his power of penetration ever so great—takes note of nothing in every individual disease, except the *changes* in the health of the body and the mind (morbid phenomena, accidents, symptoms) which can be perceived externally by means of the senses; that is to say, he notices only the deviations from a former healthy state of the diseased individual, which are felt by the patient himself, remarked by those around him and observed by the physician. All these perceptible signs represent the disease in its whole extent, that is, together they form the true and only conceivable portrait of the disease." (Organon, Par. 6.)

The tangible things which the examining physician finds in the body are not the disease, but merely its effects. It is as impossible, and therefore as futile, to try to find a disease in the hidden interior of the organism as it would be to try to find a thought by an exploration of the interior of the brain, the electricity in the interior of a dynamo, or the song in the throat of a bird. Such things are known only by their phenomena. Metaphysically considered, they may be said to subsist in the dynamic realm as substantial entities, or forces, but as such they are perceptible only to the "inner vision," through the eyes of the mind. They are "spiritually (that is, mentally) discerned." The metaphysical conception serves as an aid in the interpretation of the phenomena.

Practically, however, we do not deal with abstractions. We deal with facts and phenomena, with symptoms.

"The totality of these, its symptoms, *of this outwardly reflected picture of the internal essence of disease, that is, of the affection of the vital force,* must be the principal, or the sole means, whereby the disease can make known (its nature and) what remedy is required." (Organon, Par. 7.)

The removal of all the perceptible symptoms or phenomena of disease removes disease itself and restores health. Hahnemann thus philosophically distinguishes between disease itself and its causes, occasions, conditions, products and phenomena, and in so doing shows clearly that the sphere of homœopathy is limited primarily to the functional changes from which the phenomena of disease arise. In other words, homœopathy is confined to and operative only in the sphere of vital dynamics.

Primarily homœopathy has nothing to do with any *tangible or physical* cause, effect or product of disease, although secondarily it is related to all of them. Effects of disease in morbid function and sensation may remain after the causes have been removed. Removal of the tangible products of disease, if it be too far advanced, may have to be relegated to surgery. Homœopathy deals directly only with disease itself, the *morbid vital processes* manifested by perceptible symptoms, which may remain and continue after the causes have been removed and conditions changed.

It stands to reason, as Hahnemann says, that every intelligent physician, having a knowledge of rational etiology, will first remove by appropriate means, as far as possible, every exciting and maintaining cause of disease and obstacle to cure, and endeavor to establish a correct and orderly course of living for his patient, with due regard to mental and physical hygiene. Failing to do this, but little impression can be made by homœopathic remedies, and what slight impression is made will be of short duration.

Having done this, he addresses himself to the problem of finding that remedy, the symptoms of which in their nature, origin and order of development are most similar to the symptoms of the patient, and to the proper management of it, when found, as to size and frequency of doses.

While gross pathological tissue changes, organic lesions, morphological disproportions, neoplasms and the physical effects of mechanical causes are not primarily within the domain of *Similia,* and therefore are not the object of homœopathic treatment, the morbid processes from which they arise, or to which they lead, are amenable to homœopathic medication. Homœopathic remedies, by virtue of their power to control vital functions and increase resistance, often exercise a favorable influence upon physical development as well as upon the tangible products of disease or accident. Thus, the growth of tumors may be retarded or arrested; absorption and repair promoted, even to a total removal of the morbid product or growth; secretions and excretions may be increased or decreased; eruptions, sores and ulcers healed. But all these happy tangible results are only incidental and secondary to the real cure which takes place *solely in the functional or dynamical sphere,* quelling disturbance, controlling metabolism, antidoting poisons, raising resistance and bringing about cure by the dynamical influence of the symptomatically similar remedy.

Following the exclusion method adopted by Dake, in his "Therapeutic Methods," and using a modification of his phrasing, the sphere of *Similia* may be defined as follows:

1. Homœopathy relates primarily to no affection of health where the exciting cause of disease is constantly present and operative.

2. It relates primarily to no affections of health which will, of themselves, cease after the removal of the exciting cause by physical, chemical or hygienic measures.

3. It relates primarily to no affections of health occasioned by the injury or destruction of tissues which are incapable of restoration.

4. It relates primarily to no affections of health where the vital reactive power of the organism to medicines is exhausted, obstructed or prevented.

5. It relates to no affection of health, the symptomatic likeness of which may not be perceptibly produced in the healthy organism by medical means, nor to affections in which such symptoms are not perceptible.

The class not excluded, the one in which homœopathy is universal and paramount to all other methods, must be made up of *affections of the living organism in which perceptible symptoms exist, similar to those producible by pathogenic means, in organisms having the integrity of tissue and reactive power necessary to recovery, the exciting causes of the affections and obstacles to cure having been removed, or having ceased to be operative.*

The sphere of *Similia* in medicine is thus limited to those morbid functional conditions and processes which result primarily from the dynamic action upon the living organism of morbific agents inimical to life.

The living organism may be acted upon or affected primarily

in three ways: (1) Mechanically. (2) Chemically. (3) Dynamically. The causes of disease fall naturally under these three heads.

Under the head of mechanical causes of disease come all traumatic agencies, such as lesions, injuries and destruction of tissues resulting from physical force; morbid growths, formations and foreign substances; congenitally defective or absent organs or parts, prolapsed or displaced organs, etc. These conditions are related primarily to surgery, physical therapeutics and hygiene.

The destructive action of certain chemical poisons such as the acids and alkalies is a sufficient illustration of the chemical causes of disease, although all such agents have also secondary dynamical effects, which come within the sphere of homœopathy. Diseases arising from these causes require the use of chemical or physiological antidotes, combined in some cases with measures for the physical expulsion of the offending substances, and followed by homœopathic treatment for the functional derangements which remain or follow.

Entozoa or organized living animal parasites, when their presence in the body gives rise to disease, must be expelled by mechanical measures or by the administration of medicines capable of weakening or destroying them without endangering the person suffering from their presence. Dynamical treatment on homœopathic principles may be required to remove the functional derangements and restore the patient to health.

The effects of dynamical causes of disease, by which is meant all those intangible and medicinal or toxic agents and influences which primarily disturb the vital functions of mind and body, come legitimately within the sphere of *Similia*. These are very numerous, but they may be roughly classified as (1) mental or psychical, atmospheric, thermic, electric, telluric and climatic, (2) dietetic, hygienic, contagious, infectious and specific—the last three including all disorders arising from the use or abuse of drugs, and from all bacterial agents or pathogenic microörganisms which produce their effects through their specific toxins or alkaloids. Homœopathy successfully treats bacterial or zymotic diseases, such as cholera, yellow fever, typhus and typhoid fever, malarial fever, diphtheria, tuberculosis and pneumonia, by internal homœopathic medicines, without resorting to bactericides, germicides or antiseptics. Such agents have their use only in the field of sanitation, which is environmental, not personal. We disinfect the typhoid patient's excretions but not the patient himself.

Again quoting Dake's admirable exposition, but qualifying his third proposition, and adding a fifth paragraph:

"The domain of *Similia* may be reached by another route. Looking at the various drugs and other agencies capable of influencing health, and advancing, as before, by the method of exclusion, it may be said:

"1. The homœopathic law relates to no agents intended to affect the organism chemically.

"2. It relates to none applied for mechanical effect simply.

"3. It relates to none required in the development or support of the organism when in health.

"4. It relates to none employed directly to remove or destroy the parasites which infest or prey upon the human body.

"Looking over the armamentarium of the therapeutist for agents not excluded, one class is found, namely: *those agents which affect the organism as to health in ways not governed by chemistry, mechanics, or hygiene, but those capable of producing ailments similar to those found in the sick.*"

In regard to Dake's third proposition it can and will be shown that, inasmuch as the development and support of the organism when in health depends upon the principle of *assimilation,* as demonstrated by Fincke, the principle of *Similia* does relate to these processes; for assimilation depends upon mutual action, upon action and reaction, and this is the fundamental principle of homœopathy.

To the foregoing propositions as formulated by Dake one more should be added.

5. The homœopathic law relates to no agents or drugs administered for their direct or so-called physiological effects.

Circumstances arise occasionally which make it necessary, temporarily, for the homœopathic physician to use drugs in "physiological" (really, pathogenic) doses for their palliative effect. Although the ruling principle of his medical life is *cure by symptom-similarity,* and that end is always held in view as an ideal, he

THE SCOPE OF HOMŒOPATHY

is not thereby forbidden the use of palliative measures in cases where they are appropriate and necessary.

Hahnemann, after showing the futility of antipathic medication as a curative method, and pointing out the dangers incidental to its use, admits the utility and necessity of resorting to palliation in certain emergencies. In a note to Paragraph 67, he says:

"Only in the most urgent cases, where danger to life and imminent death allow no time for the action of a homœopathic remedy—not hours, sometimes not even quarter hours and scarcely minutes—in sudden accidents occurring to previously healthy individuals—for example, in asphyxia and suspended animation from lightning, from suffocation, freezing, drowning, etc.—it is admissible and judicious at all events as a preliminary measure, to stimulate the irritability and sensibility (the physical life), with a palliative, as for instance, with gentle electric shocks, with clysters of strong coffee, with a stimulating odor, gradual application of heat, etc. When this stimulation is effected, the play of vital organs goes on again in its former healthy manner, for there is here no disease to be removed, but merely an obstruction and suppression of the healthy vital force. To this category belong various antidotes to sudden poisonings; alkalies for mineral acids, hepar sulphuris for metallic poisons, coffee and camphor (and ipecacuanha) for poisoning by opium, etc."

The principle of palliation is here recognized and a few illustrations given of its legitimate application in one class of cases. If it is noted that all these illustrative cases are characterized by *shock*, or collapse, it will be seen that the principle has a somewhat wider application than appears on first consideration of the cases enumerated by Hahnemann. It may fairly be extended, for example, to cover certain cases where sudden and unendurable pain occurs and collapse is threatened by such semi-mechanical conditions as the presence or passage of renal calculi and gravel, or biliary concretions. In exceptional cases of these and similar conditions, analgesics may be used temporarily as anæsthetics are used in surgical and dental operations, and for the same purpose, that is, to prevent or relieve shock.

When all has been said and the scope of homœopathy has been defined as clearly as possible, it is evident that there is a borderland between homœopathy and its related sciences around which it is impossible to draw sharp lines of demarcation. In this region each physician must be governed by his own individual judgment and the circumstances of the case. It follows that there will always be differences of opinion between individual physicians under such circumstances. The physician who is imbued with the spirit of homœopathy endeavors always to keep his mind open and free from prejudice. While striving always to perfect his knowledge of homœopathic technic in order that he may meet any emergency and extend the borders of his art to the farthest limits, he never forgets that the necessities and the welfare of his patient are first. He will not allow either pride or prejudice to obscure his sense of his own limitations, nor those of his art. Circumstances sometimes arise when the strongest man and ablest prescriber, by reason of the great moral pressure brought to bear upon him by the peculiarities of his patient, of the environment, or from lack of time, will be compelled to tide over a period of unendurable suffering by the use of analgesics, or of some other measure to meet extraordinary emergencies. He does this as a charitable concession to the weakness of human nature, his own perhaps as well as others, without in the least degree lowering his standards, or bringing discredit upon himself or his art. He does this knowing, perhaps, that if he had time and the circumstances permitted, he could do better. But time and circumstances are sometimes, at least temporarily, beyond his control. It is possible to violate the *spirit* by adhering too closely to the *letter* of the law. Victory is sometimes gained by appearing to yield, which is quite in accord with the principle of *Similia,* a sort of moral homœopathy. A strategic retreat to another line of defense in war often gives a stronger base from which to launch a successful attack.

In cases of renal or hepatic colic, for example: If the physician is firm and calm as well as skillful, and possesses the entire confidence of the patient and his family and friends, he may be able to alleviate the agonizing pain and carry such cases through to a happy termination by the use of homœopathic remedies alone. It has often been done and, when possible, is the ideal way

But the physician may have been newly called to the case or family and not have had time to gain their complete confidence by the results of his work and teaching. Patients have to be educated in the principles and methods of homœopathy by discussion, instruction and demonstration, and this requires time. When they have felt or witnessed the results of competent homœopathic prescribing they acquire confidence. Some become enthusiastic advocates and propagandists of homœopathy, and are always ready to uphold and coöperate with their physician in demonstrating its methods even in the gravest emergencies. Others are interested only in quick results, caring little or nothing about how they are obtained. The latter are very difficult to hold in such cases and some of them will not continue with the conscientious homœopathician, no matter what he does. Between these two classes exists a third, the members of which can be interested in homœopathy to a degree that will enable the practitioner to hold them as patients and retain their confidence and coöperation in homœopathic treatment in all but extreme cases. It is in such cases that the pressure referred to will be brought to bear upon him, and he may be compelled to resort temporarily to palliation to gain time and strengthen his position. Unless he can do this there is but one honorable course left for him to pursue—resign the case and withdraw. In pursuing either of those courses the conscientious practitioner is beyond the criticism of all fair-minded persons. But he is always open and frequently subjected to the attacks of prejudice, bigotry and jealousy, and to these the best defense is silence and a clear conscience.

CHAPTER V

THE UNITY OF MEDICINE

"As our studies in medicine penetrate deeper into the problems of each individual branch or specialty one fact stands out with ever-increasing emphasis; namely, that medicine is a unit and incapable of real division into specialties. The superior man in medicine of the future will not be the great laboratory worker, or the man who is known for his studies in metabolism, or the expert gastro-enterologist or neurologist or surgeon, or he who stands preëminently above his confreres in his knowledge of diseases of the heart and arterial system or of the lungs, *but the man who recognizes the fact that the truths derived from all these sources of study and investigation must be interpreted as belonging to the patient as a whole*—in other words, *the internist who appreciates the unity of medicine.* The distinguished specialist will be one who regards his field of study in its intimate relationships to *the body as a whole.*"

With these weighty words, Francis Marion Pottenger, A. M., M. D., LL. D., F. A. C. P., the most distinguished specialist in diseases of the chest in the United States, opens his great book entitled "Symptoms of Visceral Disease."

Mistaken ideals, wrong theories, wrong practice, materialism, commercialism and selfish competition, as well as the great enlargement of the field of medicine in the advance of science, have led to overspecialization in the medical profession, the disappearance of the general practitioner and the springing up of numerous so-called "non-medical" cults and fads.

The Genius of Homœopathy.—There are "57 different varieties" of specialists—one for almost every organ of the body, besides those who deal with many other subjects connected with medicine. In addition to the old-time allopathic, homœopathic and eclectic schools (which are still with us) we now have the pharmico-physio-mechano-electro-hydro-balneo-sero-vaccino and radiotherapeutic schools, not to mention the osteopaths, the chiropractors, the Christian Scientists and the mental, psychic and spiritual healers, all of whom are "practicing medicine" in the broad sense of the term.

There is an old saying: "It takes nine tailors to make a man." Now we might say: "It takes nine specialists to make a physician," if it were not that nine would not be enough to make a good, all-around physician of the old school.

The people realize, in a blind sort of way, that they are getting from the medical profession a good many things they do not want, and are not getting some very important things which they need. The failure of the surgeon and organ specialists to do more than palliate or remove the tangible products of disease; the rise of the seductive serum and vaccine therapy, and the reign of the reptilean derived hypodermic needle; the disappearance of the general practitioner with the system of medical education which made him, and the refusal of the profession to accept the beneficent law of therapeutic medication and its corrollaries enunciated by Hahnemann, are the main reasons for the increase of quackery and humbug in the practice of medicine and the rise of non-medical cults. There is rebellion and revolution in the medical world as well as in all the other worlds.

Are we really any better off by all the elaborate specialization in medicine? In certain respects, perhaps, yes. In general, no. A reasonable amount of specialization in medicine, as in other professions, is necessary and beneficial. Medicine covers a very broad field. It is too great to be compassed by the activities of any individual, except in a broad way. The exigencies of the situation require that it should be divided into certain departments, any one of which is large enough to fully engage the time, talents and energy of one man. But no man can successfully do the work of a department without recognizing the essential unity of medicine and the vital relation of his chosen department to every other department. Especially is this true of the internist—the individual who devotes himself to curative medicine as distinguished from preventive medicine and surgery; and still more is it true of the pharmaco-therapeutist who relies mainly for his results upon the scientific use of drugs, as in the case of the homœopathician, who is legitimately a specialist under the same rules as govern any other legitimate specialist.

The vital, organic relation between all the departments of medicine must never be overlooked. The science of medicine exists only in order that the art of medicine may be made effectual in the prevention, amelioration and cure of disease. The specialties in medicine are of little value in the treatment of disease unless they are correlated and directed in their application by the internist —the general practitioner—who views and treats every case as a whole. All the surgery, all the organ specializing, all the theorizing, laboratory research, classifying, naming and explaining of diseases amount to very little if it does not lead to the cure of the patient.

Now cure relates to the case as a whole, not merely to a part or an organ. A human being is something more than a miscellaneous assortment of eyes, ears, nose, throat, lungs, etc.—organs which the ordinary specialists, if left to themselves, usually treat as if they were independent of each other. They are only parts of a very intricate machine—the most intricate machine in the world. They are assembled according to a wonderful plan made by The Designer of The Universe for the purpose of utilizing the divine power of life. Life, the motive power, flows through them all and unites them into an organic whole. Each part depends upon every other part, and all act together as one, in health or disease. All diseases originate as a disturbance of the life principle. No organ can become diseased without a preceding disturbance of the life principle in which all the other organs participate.

The cure of disease takes place in the same way. The curative remedy, through the media of the nerves and blood vessels, acts first upon the life principle everywhere present in the organism, and then upon the affected parts, in a perfectly natural manner. It is only necessary that the remedy shall be correctly selected, properly prepared and administered by the natural channels in appropriate dosage in order to get its curative effects. No hypodermic needle is required. One who knows how to do these things never makes the mistake of treating a part as if it stood alone. Before his mental eye is always pictured the individual patient—the case as a whole.

It is a characteristic of homœopathy that all of its practical processes are governed by the principle of individualization. In its drug provings; its study of the materia medica compiled from those provings; its examination of a patient and study of a case; its selection of the remedy and its conduct of whatever auxiliary treatment is required, it seeks always to individualize.

Homœopathy recognizes the individuality of each drug and substance in nature. Its method of testing or "proving" drugs upon the healthy is designed and used for the express purpose of bringing out the symptomatic individuality of each drug so that its full powers and relations may be established. There are no "succodanæ" in the homœopathic materia medica. A given drug is symptomatically indicated in a case or it is not. There are no substitutes for the conscientious prescriber. Symptomatic comparison between similar drugs is instituted and carried on until one (the one bearing the closest symptom-similarity to the case) stands clearly out as the indicated remedy.

Homœopathy recognizes the individuality of each patient or case. The entire examination of a patient is conducted with a view to discovering not only the general or common features of the case by which it may be classified diagnostically and pathologically, but the special and particular symptoms which differentiate the case from others of the same general class. It recognizes the fact that no two cases or patients, even with the same disease, are exactly alike, and maintains that a true science of therapeutics must enable the practitioner to recognize these differences and find the needed remedy for each individual. In actual practice the "differences" are very often the deciding factor in the choice of the remedy. To use a frequently quoted epigram: "Homœopathy does not treat disease. It treats patients." In one word, it individualizes. It may be added that homœopathy is the only method by which the prescriber is able to thus individualize his medication.

In the auxiliary treatment the same principle is applied as far as possible. In dietetics, for example, instead of laying down rigid rules and making up a diet list composed of articles selected solely for their supposed chemical or physiological relation to the case, the patient's idiosyncrasies, his likes and dislikes, his aggravations and ameliorations, as revealed by his symptoms, are considered and allowed for. Nature as thus revealed in the patient's temperament, constitution and clinical history is consulted.

This is not to say that theoretical considerations are of no use or value, but simply that theory is to be checked up and modified by facts as revealed in the individual. That a patient ought to take or avoid a certain article of food does not always mean that he can do so. Frequently he can not do so. Knowledge of homœopathic principles and methods thus enables the practitioner to make these individual adjustments and modifications intelligently and overcome obstacles otherwise insurmountable.

The question of individual susceptibility to medicinal action must be considered. Susceptibility to medicinal influence varies in different individuals according to time and circumstances, as well as to different drugs. In health one may be susceptible to the action of a medicine at one time and under certain circumstances and not at other times and under other circumstances. Moreover, one may be constitutionally susceptible to only a few medicines. In sickness, susceptibility to the symptomatically similar, potentiated medicine is greatly increased, but in that case the action is curative, although new symptoms (proving) may arise if the potency be not suitable or too many doses be taken.

Age, sex, temperament and constitution; occupation, habits, climate, season, weather; the nature, type, extent and stage of the disease—everything, in fact, which modifies the psychological, physiological, or pathological status of the individual patient modifies, at the same time, the susceptibility to medicine, increasing or decreasing it, in health and disease. All these modifying factors must be observed, considered, weighed, and their influence estimated in conducting a proving, or treating a case. One will react only to a high potency, another only to a medium potency, or still another only to a low potency or tangible doses of the crude drug.

In practice, the whole scale of potencies from the lowest to the highest, is open to the homœopathic physician. He defines his power and sphere of influence over health and disease largely by the number of differing potencies he possesses and the skill with which he uses them.

Success in homœopathic treatment largely depends, therefore, upon the ability to correctly measure the individual patient's degree of susceptibility to medication and select the most appropriate potency.

Therapeutic Nihilism.—Although it has spread to all parts of the civilized world, numbering its practitioners by thousands and its patients by millions, homœopathy has never found open and general acceptance in the medical profession. Occasional conversions of individuals from the ranks of the dominant school have apparently made little impression on the profession as a whole, but the influence of Hahnemannian principles is increasingly perceptible as time goes on. By long, tedious, circuitous routes medical science appears to be approaching the goal attained over a century ago by Hahnemann.

It is only another illustration of the fact that poets, prophets and philosophers often perceive great truths and announce them to the world long before slow-moving scientists succeed in proving them to their own satisfaction.

Intuition, the highest faculty of the human mind, wings its aerial way home, while research and investigation laboriously plod their way along upon the ground.

The main subjects of controversy in the past have been: 1. The idea of a general principle of curative medication; 2, the doctrine of potentiation and the minimum dose; 3, proving medicines on the healthy, and 4, the single remedy.

Refusing to submit these questions to the test of competent, systematic investigation and experimentation, and baffled in their own efforts to find a successful way of treating the sick by medication, leaders of the dominant school have practically abandoned drugs, and now rely mainly upon surgery and hygienic methods, supplemented more recently by the use of sera and vaccines.

In pathology and physiology there has been a gradual breaking away from the tyranny of authority that has so long held the medical profession in its grip. But in pharmaco-therapy this nihilistic tendency has carried them almost to the point of complete negation.

Osler, writing in 1901, said: "He is the best physician who knows the worthlessness of most medicine."

Barker, his successor at Johns Hopkins, says: "The deathblow came first to polypharmacy. To-day with many, pharmacotherapy as a whole is almost moribund."

Billings, in his address as president of the American Medical Association, says: "Drugs, with the exception of quinine in malaria, and mercury in syphilis, are valueless as cures."

Musser, of Philadelphia, two years later, from the same chair said: "One sees less and less of the use of drugs."

Cabot, of Harvard, in his notable address before the Boston Homœopathic Medical Society, said: "I doubt if you gentlemen realize how large a proportion of our patients are treated without any drugs at all, and how little faith we have to-day in the curative power of drugs."

These extracts indicate the extremity to which some keen observers, clear thinkers and honest men of the dominant school have been driven, in the absence of a general principle of therapeutic medication. In the meantime the rank and file have gone on stolidly in the same old course of pernicious drugging.

Blinded by professional pride and prejudice, the dominant school as a whole has bitterly antagonized or ignored the principle enunciated by Hahnemann a century ago and demonstrated by him and his successors continuously ever since.

In no profession, perhaps, has there been so little open-mindedness, so little of the impersonal, so little of the true scientific spirit, as in medicine. Few indeed have there been in either school who could rise above the petty personal and professional jealousies which have hampered them into the freedom of the higher, impersonal realm of pure science. The controversial rather than the scientific spirit has ruled too largely on both sides.

In one respect, at least, the leaders of the old school are in perfect accord with the followers of Hahnemann who have always maintained that the use of drugs in the treatment of disease, except in minimum doses and in accordance with the law of similars, is both useless and injurious.

One of the first and most important truths taught to homœopathic students is that drugs, in crude form and ordinary so-called physiological doses, have the power to make even well people sick. It is demonstrated by the pathogenetic record of every drug in our materia medica. How much more injurious drugs are to sick persons, with their lower power of resistance and increased irritability, might easily be inferred theoretically if the comparative mortality rates did not continually furnish proof of their deadly influence and make such inferences superfluous.

There have been signs of a beginning change of base in the ranks of the dominant school of medicine within the last few years. Among others, the wide acceptance and practice of serum and vaccine-therapy and the hospitality of many of its advocates to the suggestion that the underlying principle of this form of treatment is analogous to, if indeed it be not in fact the homœopathic principle, tends to show a more tolerant spirit toward the idea of a general therapeutic principle governing the curative action of all drugs in all diseases by medication.

General medicine has made great advances since the days of Hahnemann; notably in the sciences of biology, physiology, pathology and bacteriology. Research and discovery in these fields have revealed facts which not only tend to confirm, but to elucidate the essential principles of homœopathy. This has not escaped the notice of certain of the leaders in the dominant school of medicine, although for obvious reasons they prefer not to enlarge upon it publicly. Having made and announced an important discovery in medical science, it is not flattering to one's vanity to be shown that in all essential points the same discovery was made, announced and put to use in a better way more than a century ago, by one who has been held up to obloquy and scorn by a large part of the profession ever since.

Modern biological science has confirmed homœopathists anew in their belief that in homœopathy they have not only the basic law of therapeutic medication, but also of all tissue reaction. Study of the reactions of protoplasm to stimuli (chemical, electrical and mechanical) has led to the formulation of the biological law now universally accepted, viz: *"The same agent which in relatively large quantities damages or destroys activity, will in relatively small quantities stimulate it."*

This is substantially a statement of the well-known law upon which homœopathy is based. It establishes a firm foundation for a practical system of therapeutic medication formulated by the methods of pure experimental science. It leads naturally and logically to systematic experimentation with drugs upon healthy, living subjects to determine their natural tissue relations and organic affinities and the kind of reactions their administration arouses.

Reactions in the living subject manifest themselves in perceptible functional and tissue changes which, in the case of human beings, may be felt and intelligently observed, described, measured and recorded. In medical parlance, reactions are expressed by symptoms, subjectively and objectively. Under this principle and by this method have our homœopathic provings been conducted, and from these provings our materia medica is constructed.

Tests, of course, are conducted with doses only sufficient to arouse characteristic reactions without endangering or destroying life, since to do otherwise would defeat the end in view.

Knowing experimentally the damaging or pathogenetic effects of relatively large doses of a drug upon the healthy living subject; knowing also that relatively small doses of the same drug exercise a more moderate and stimulating effect, the next logical step is to determine the natural relation between drugs and disease.

Systemic reactions to pathogenetic agents of every kind, tangible or intangible, are observed and studied by the physician in the light of this principle in the same manner as the reactions of protoplasm to drugs and other stimuli are studied by the biologist; for the physician is essentially a biologist, as medicine is fundamentally a biological science.

Systemic reactions to morbific influences, pathogenic organisms and drugs alike are all manifested by perceptible phenomena or symptoms. In fact, the student of the comparative symptomatology of drugs and diseases needs not to progress very far to realize that it is impossible to draw any sharp line of demarcation between them. All diseases are produced by morbific agencies or poisons of some kind, primarily or secondarily generated, and the symptoms of disease are precisely similar to the symptoms of drugs. It is not illogical to deduce that the direct causative agents are similar, if not identical, and that the differences in effects are due to differences in the size and quantity of the doses, the morphological peculiarities of the subjects and different conditions.

Modern medicine in its use of the sera and vaccines, is demonstrating the identity, or at least the similarity, of disease-producing and disease-curing agents, and in so doing is demonstrating the homœopathic principle.

The biological law under discussion brings again to the front, as of fundamental importance, the old, old subject of The Dose, which has received so much discussion in the past. Perhaps from this time on the discussion can be carried on without bigotry, acrimony or prejudice to a point where the two schools of medicine can arrive at some amicable understanding based upon the acceptance of a general principle of therapeutic medication.

Medical Sciolists.—The homœopathic medical profession would have been spared a large part of the tiresome and unprofitable discussions which have wasted time, paper and printer's ink in the past if would-be critics, before entering the literary field, had at least informed themselves correctly of the derivation and meaning of certain terms used by those whom they attacked. Misunderstanding or misusing a word, they attached an arbitrary or imaginary meaning to it and proceeded to belabor their "man of straw."

In reviewing the controversial literature of homœopathy it is surprising to find so large a part of it thus initiated. Much of it could never have been written by men who had even "a speaking acquaintance" with sciences other than the one they professed to represent.

Men who thoroughly understand a subject rarely misunderstand each other. They have been over the same course and learned the same language. They know the groundwork and essentials of their common art or science, and they also know something of its relations with other branches of art and science.

All true sciences are interrelated. They touch one another at many points. Each is dependent upon the others in many respects. They often "exchange works" as well as words.

Entrance upon the profession of medicine has, until recent years, been so easy and unrestricted, that a large proportion of its matriculants had not even the equivalent of a modern grammar school education. With little or none of the cultural and still less of the scientific training which goes into the make-up of a well educated man, they have been permitted to take a course in medicine and enter upon its practice. Innate ability, a studious disposition and hard work have enabled some of these men to make up for their pre-medical shortcomings and earn high honors; but the majority have been medical misfits, without whom the profession and the public would have been better off.

So long as such men confined their attention strictly to the practice of medicine, according to their lights, much could be forgiven. But when they invaded the literary field and began to write of matters of which they knew little or nothing, and even to set themselves up as critics of men who did know, patience ceased to be a virtue. In pillorizing the culprits, the editors of magazines and society Transactions who admitted such trash to their pages should not be overlooked. Verily, they have much to answer for!

A striking example of the misunderstanding and misuse of words is found in the voluminous and for a long time seemingly endless discussion centered around the word "spiritual," used by Hahnemann in paragraph 9 of the Organon, which reads as follows: "In the healthy condition of man, the *spiritual* vital force ('autocracy), the dynamis that animates the material body (organism) rules with unbounded sway, and retains all the parts of both sensations and functions, so that our in-dwelling, reason-gifted mind can freely employ this living, healthy instrument for the higher purposes of our existence."

Failing to see that Hahnemann had permissibly used the word "spiritual" as the antithesis of the words "material" or "tangible," the would-be critics swooped down upon it like a hawk upon a chicken, fastened their talons in it and proceeded to make the feathers fly. Unfamiliar also with the word "dynamis," and ignorant of its derivation and meaning, they turned their imagination loose and assumed that Hahnemann was referring to some mystical, "spiritualistic" sort of a thing which to their half-educated and crudely materialistic minds had no existence. Much ridicule and cheap wit, as well as invective, were wasted upon Hahnemann and homœopathy.

Had they taken pains to refer to any good dictionary they might have learned that dynamis is a Greek noun meaning power or force; the power or principle *objectively considered,* applied by Hahnemann to the life principle.

By the use of that word and its adjectives, dynamic and dynamical (of or pertaining to forces not in equilibrium; pertaining to motion as the result of force; opposed to static) Hahnemann introduces us into the realm of Dynamics, the science which treats of the motion of bodies and action of forces in producing or changing their motion. In medicine dynamical commonly refers to functional as opposed to organic disease. Hahnemann thus opened the way for bringing homœopathy under mathematical laws, creating the Science of Homœopathics and giving it its rightful place in the "Circle of the Sciences."

CHAPTER VI

Life, Health and Disease

Life is the invisible, substantial, intelligent, individual, co-ordinating power and cause directing and controlling the forces involved in the production and activity of any organism possessing individuality.

Health is that balanced condition of the living organism in which the integral, harmonious performance of the vital functions tends to the preservation of the organism and the normal development of the individual.

Disease is an abnormal vital process, a changed condition of life, which is inimical to the true development of the individual and tends to organic dissolution.

Vital phenomena in health and disease are caused by the reaction of the vital substantial power or principle of the organism to various external stimuli. So long as a healthy man lives normally in a favorable environment he moves, feels, thinks, acts and reacts in an orderly manner. If he violates the laws of life, or becomes the victim of an unfavorable environment, disorder takes the place of order, dis-ease destroys ease, he suffers and his body deteriorates.

When organic vitality is exhausted, or is withdrawn, his transient material organism dies, yields to chemical laws and is dissolved into its elements, while his substantial, spiritual organism continues its existence in a higher realm.

Agents, material or immaterial, which modify health or cause disease, act solely by virtue of their own substantial, entitative existence and the co-existence of the vital substance, which reacts in the living organism to every impression made from within or without. The dead body reacts only to physical and chemical agents, under the action of which it is reduced to its chemical elements and dissipated as a material organism.

All reactions to stimuli by which the functions and activities of the living body are carried on, originate in the primitive life substance at the point where it becomes materialized as cells and protoplasmic substance.

Agents from without which affect the living body to produce changes and modifications of its functions and sensations, act upon the protoplasm through the medium of the brain and nervous system. Food, drink, heat, light, air, electricity and drugs, as well as mental stimuli, all act primarily upon the living substance as materialized in the cells of the central nervous system, calling forth the reactions which are represented by functions and sensations.

"Power resides at the center, and from the center of power, force flows."

The phenomena of life, as manifested in growth, nutrition, repair, secretion, excretion, self-recognition, self-preservation and reproduction, all take their direction from an originating center. From the lowest cell to the highest and most complex organism, this principle holds true. Cell wall and protoplasmic contents develop from the central nucleus, and that from the centrosome, which is regarded as the "center of force" in the cell. All fluids, tissues and organs develop from the cell from within outwards, from center to circumference.

Organic control is from the center. In the completely developed human organism vital action is controlled from the central nervous system. The activities of the cell are controlled from the centrosome, which may be called the brain of the cell.

The central nervous system may be compared to a dynamo. As a dynamo is a machine, driven by steam or some other force, which, through the agency of electro-magnetic induction from a surrounding magnetic field, converts into electrical energy in the form of current the mechanical energy expended upon it, so the central nervous system is a machine driven by chemical force derived from food which, through the agency of electro-vital induction from a surrounding vital field, converts into vital energy. in the form of nerve current or impulses, the chemico-physical energy expended upon it.

As an electrical transportation system depends for its working force upon the dynamo located in its central power station, so the human body depends for the force necessary to carry on its operations upon the central power station, located in the central nervous system.

Any disturbance of conditions at the central power station is immediately manifested externally at some point in the system; and any injury to or break in the external system is immediately reflected back to the central station.

In health and disease it is the same, both being essentially merely conditions of life in the living organism, convertible each into the other. In each condition the modifying agent or factor acts primarily upon the internal life principle, which is the living substance of the organism. This reacts and produces external phenomena through the medium of the brain and nervous system which extends to every part of the body. Food or poison, toxins or antitoxins, therapeutic agents or pathogenic micro-organisms, all act upon and by virtue of the existence of the reacting life principle or living substance of the organism.

Cure of disease, or the restoration of health, likewise begins at the center and spreads outwardly, the symptoms disappearing from within outward, from above downward and in the reverse order of their appearance.

Resistance to morbific agents is from the center where life reigns. Vital resistance is the defensive reaction of living substance to noxious elements and organisms and to disease-producing causes and agents in general, in obedience to the inherent instinct or law of self-preservation, which belongs to life in organism.

Metaphorically speaking, disease is resistance. Disease, manifested by symptoms, expresses the vital reaction and resistance of the living organism to the inroads of some injurious agent or influence. It is a battle, a struggle, a costly and painful resistance to an invader.

Strictly speaking, it is not against disease that we struggle, but against the causes of disease. The actual causes of disease, in the last analysis, are from without. They do not exist in the life substance itself. They are "foreign to the spirit," to man's true nature. They become operative or effective in the organism conditionally, by virtue of the existence of the vital principle of susceptibility, reaction and resistance, and of a living organism in and through which action and reaction can take place.

Matter and Force.—Physical science declares that matter

is indestructible. Matter is corporeal substance; the form of being or substance that is characterized by extension, inertia, weight, etc., or, in general, by the properties cognized by the senses. The constitution and mode of production of matter are traced backward from mass through molecules, atoms, and electrons to a vibratory or radiant state of matter supposed to exist in the interatomic ether of space.

Ether is a hypothetical medium filling all space, through which, in the form of transverse wave-motion, radiant or vibratory energy of all kinds, including light-waves, is propagated. According to physical science, all energy exists in the ether, and matter may be regarded as, in a sense, a condensation, "a specifically modified form of ether," as Lodge puts it. This is as far as physical science can go. Of the nature and source of the "Energy," in other words, of *what it is* that radiates through the ether in the form of "transverse waves," physical science can tell us nothing. In stating this conception science tacitly admits the substantial character of the ether, or energy in general, and of specific forms of energy in particular, although its phraseology is often vague and its terms contradictory. Physical science does, however, adhere to the general principles of the indestructibility of matter and the persistence of force. It is thus far in harmony with the more advanced position taken in the substantial philosophy. It is much to have arrived at that point in thinking. But of incorporeal living substance, or Life and Mind and Intelligence as the primary source and basis of all energy, current science has as yet only a faint conception; although more than one physical scientist has reached the conclusion that, in the last analysis, all force is a manifestation of Will, and that every physical action is primarily a psychical action.

Biological science traces matter backward from organism through cells, nuclei, to the centrosome, an organ found in the protoplasm, but usually only occurring in close connection with the nucleus. When active the centrosome is said to be "at the center of a sphere of attraction and a system of rays," and is regarded as the dynamic center governing karyokinesis and cell division.

Biological science, therefore, when examined closely is found to recognize, at least tacitly, the existence of Life as a substantial, entitative, indestructible power. How or by what else could the vital force necessary to carry on vital processes be generated? How else could there be in the cell a "dynamic center?" Dynamic center means "center of power." Statically, power means capacity of a person or thing for work, for producing the force by which work is done. There must be a source from which force is produced or drawn, and that source must be substantial. Kinetically, power is the cause, force the medium, and work the effect. Power, therefore, considered either as an attribute or the thing itself, is actually a substantial, entitative being.

Since life can come only from life, biological science, in thus placing the centrosome at the center of "a sphere of attraction," places it in a surrounding field of what can only be *incorporeal living substance,* from which alone could it attract the wherewithal to construct the cell and endow it with the functions of organization, growth and reproduction.

As the active agent and center of attraction the centrosome is a medium, standing between the field of life on the one side, and the field of matter on the other side, acting under the law of attraction or affinity, by means of which vital force is drawn from the surrounding vital field and converted or transformed into the physical or chemical force which acts directly upon the matter of which the cell is composed. The centrosome also, like the central nervous system, may be compared in this respect to a dynamo, which acts in a similar manner in the conversion of mechanical energy into electric energy or current.

Biological science as yet is neither explicit nor comprehensive in this matter. It places the centrosome "at the center of a field of attraction," but does not define or enumerate all the contents of that field. Enumerating only the physical or chemical forces and the various forms of matter of which the cell is composed, it implies that these are all the field contains. Biology, the science of life and living things, thus evades the acknowledgment of Life as a specific power, principle or substance, and defines it merely as *a state* of the organism, *a condition;* or as arising out of physical and chemical elements and forces acting so as to result in some unexplained way in the evolution of the individual living beings and the development of the species.

Such a definition fails to explain some of the most important phenomena of living organisms, such as growth, reproduction, self-repair and constant changes with continued identity (not to speak of consciousness, feeling and thought), because it leaves out Life, the most important element of all. It is like the play of Hamlet with Hamlet left out.

It is an axiom of biological science that life comes only from preceding life.

The surrounding field of "the sphere of attraction," at the center of which biology places the centrosome, must therefore contain the life substance as well as the matter of which the cell is composed upon which the attraction is exerted.

Attraction is a force exercised mutually upon each other by two or more bodies, particles or substances, tending to make them approach each other, or to prevent their separating.

As the active agent or center of attraction the centrosome is a medium, standing between life on the one side and matter on the other side.

The central nervous system, made up of innumerable cells, with their nuclei and centrosomes, has already been compared to a dynamo. So each individual cell with its nucleus and centrosome may be called a dynamo in miniature. A dynamo is essentially a converter of one form of energy into another. Standing at the center of the field of attraction and acting in all directions under the law of attraction, the centrosome, through the agency of induction from the surrounding vital field, converts the chemical energy derived from nutrient matter into vital energy.

In no other way and from no other source could the centrosome attract that ruling element by which the living human body and brain are endowed with their peculiar properties and functions of organization, growth, self-repair, reproduction, intelligence, reason, feeling and will.

Electrical science, in its theory of electro-magnetic induction and conversion, has thus paved the way for a clearer understanding of the *modus operandi* of the life principle.

Physics and biology are in harmony with homœopathics, the science of homœopathy. Their basic principles are identical. The respective scientific explanations of the origin, constitution and transformation of matter and the laws governing the same agree perfectly as far as they go.

The explanations of physics and biology serve equally well for homœopathy in its physical and biological aspects. Ionization, for example, the breaking apart of electrolytes into anions and cations by solution or other process, chemical or mechanical (the theory of electrolytic dissociation) is an adequate physical explanation of what occurs in the preparation by trituration, solution and dilution according to scale of homœopathic high potencies. The much-derided and discussed "infinitesimals" of homœopathy are found at last, in the farthest advance of science, to be "common property," under the general mathematical "Theory of Infinitesimals." Physicists and biologists, as well as homœopathists, have been led to the adoption of the theory of the infinitesimal to explain their phenomena, and of the infinitesimal quantity to accomplish their ends.

The amazing achievements of modern physical, chemical and electrical science have been made possible only by knowledge of the powers, properties and laws of the infinitesimal.

Mathematics, greatest and most ancient of the sciences, opened the way with its Infinitesimal Differential and Integral Calculus, and laid the foundation upon which later coming sciences were built—homœopathy among them.

The Nature of Disease.—It has been said of homœopathy that it is "not a theory of disease, but a theory of cure." It is a taking phrase, but like many other such epigrams it embodies only a half truth, and half truths are fatal to right thinking. It can easily be proved by reference to the writings of Hahnemann that a theory of disease lies at the very foundation of homœopathy. This theory, based upon the general philosophical conception of the unity, universality and supremacy of Life and Mind, out of which grew Hahnemann's physio-dynamical doctrine of the life force, was an anticipation by more than eighty years of the biological theory propounded in 1897 by Virchow, the great German pathologist.

Virchow's Cellular Pathology, in which he summed up his long lifetime of research and study, was until recently the highest medical authority on the subject. Virchow reached the conclusion that "pathology is but a branch of biology; that is, that disease is merely life under altered conditions." This conclusion was hailed as "the most important achievement of the nineteenth century" and to Virchow, in recognition thereof, almost royal honors were granted.

Eighty-four years before Virchow published his famous dictum, namely, in 1813, Hahnemann, in his "Spirit of the Homœopathic Doctrine" and elsewhere in his writings, used the following expressions: "To the explanation of human life, as also its two-fold conditions, health and disease, the principles by which we explain other phenomena are quite inapplicable." Again he says: "Now as the condition of the organism and its health state depends solely on the state of life which animates it, in like manner it follows that the altered state, which we term disease, consists in a condition altered originally only in its vital sensibilities and functions, irrespective of all chemical or mechanical principles; in short, it must consist in an altered dynamical condition, a changed mode of being, whereby a change in the properties of the material component parts of the body is afterward affected, which is a necessary consequence of the morbidly altered condition of the living whole in every individual case."

"Disease will not cease to be (spiritual) dynamic aberrations of our spiritlike life, manifested by sensations and actions, that is, they will not cease to be immaterial modifications of our sensorial condition (health)."

Thus, in terms almost identical with those of his great compatriot, Hahnemann stated the present accepted biological conception of disease, and in so stating it anticipated, by nearly a century, one of the profoundest conclusions of modern scientific thought.

There are other subjects in which Hahnemann, by marvelous foresight and intuition, anticipated the conclusions of modern science. Among them were certain of the discoveries of Koch and Pasteur.

In 1883 Koch was sent by the German government on a special mission to India to study Asiatic cholera. He discovered and was able to demonstrate the presence, in the intestines of cholera patients, of a spiral, threadlike bacterium which readily breaks up into little curved segments like a comma, each less than 1/10,000 of an inch in length. These microscopical living organisms multiply with great rapidity and swarm by the million in the intestines of such patients. Koch showed that they can be cultivated artificially in dilute gelatine broth and obtained in spoonfuls. He also showed that cholera could be produced in animals by administering to them a pure, concentrated culture of these germs, although it was only done with great difficulty after many experiments. He therefore held that the germs were the cause of cholera.

Other investigators, however, for a time failed to duplicate his results and refused to accept Koch's conclusion. Pettenkofer, of Munich, who did not believe that the comma bacillus was the effective cause of cholera, to prove his contention, bravely swallowed a whole spoonful of the cultivated germs. His assistants did the same and none suffered any ill effect. This somewhat spectacular demonstration did not impress others, however, many of whom realized that it must be necessary for the human intestine to be in a favorable or susceptible condition, an unhealthy condition, for the bacillus to thrive and multiply in it.

A little later Metchnikoff of Paris repeated Pettenkofer's experiment. He swallowed a cultivated mass of the bacili on three successive days and had no injurious result. Others in his laboratory did the same with the result of only a slight intestinal disurbance. But of a dozen who thus put the matter to the proof in the Pasteur Institute, *one individual* acquired an attack of the Indian cholera which very nearly caused his death. That put an end to such experiments and conclusively demonstradted that Koch's comma bacillus is really capable of producing true cholera, *when right conditions exist*.

The announcement of Koch's discovery made a furore in the medical world. Glowing hopes of cure were based upon it, soon, alas! to be disappointed. It seemed such a simple proposition in those days: "Kill the germs and cure the disease!" At last cholera was to be "stamped out!"

It was very easy to kill the germs—in a test tube; but to kill them in the living organism of the cholera patient without killing the patient was quite a different proposition, as they very soon learned. In spite of all attempts at cure based upon such crude reasoning, cholera continued its ravages with undiminished mortality. Now hear what Hahnemann said more than fifty years before all this happened.

When Asiatic cholera invaded Europe in 1831 and began ravaging the population, it was realized that it was of the utmost importance to learn its modes of propagation and extension. Hufeland, the great leader of medical thought in Europe at that period, believed and taught that cholera was of atmospheric-telluric origin, from which there could be no protection. Against this awful error Hahnemann protested in a vigorous essay on "The Mode of Propagation of the Asiatic Cholera," in which he held that it was *"communicable by contagion only, and propagated from one individual to another."* Illustrating and explaining its mode of origin and propagation he says: "On board ships, in those confined spaces, filled with mouldy, watery vapors, the cholera miasm finds a favorable element for its multiplication, and grows into an enormously increased brood of those *excessively minute, invisible, living creatures,* so inimical to human life, of which the contagious matter of the cholera most probably consists." He refers again and again to "the invisible cloud" that hovers around those who have been in contact with the disease, "composed of probably millions of these miasmatic *animated beings,* which, at first developed on the broad marshy banks of the tepid Ganges, always search out the human being."

Consider this amazing statement in which Hahnemann again, by more than half a century, anticipates the conclusions and demonstrations of modern science.

Remember, Hahnemann had no microscope. That instrument, except in its crude form as a magnifying glass, used as a sort of plaything, did not exist. His conclusion was a deduction of pure reason from observed facts, which he states at some length in his essay. Moreover, Hahnemann by an exercise of that same thinking faculty which his wise old father had so carefully trained in his childhood and youth in the old home in Meissen, also discovered and announced the true curative remedies for the disease and that before he had ever personally seen a case.

It was reserved for Koch, who had a microscope, to demonstrate ocularly the absolute truth of Hahnemann's idea. Whether

Koch had read the writings of Hahnemann on this subject is open to question. They were published in book form and were to be found on the shelves of any great library, accessible to all students. If Koch and Pasteur had read and were familiar with the teaching of Hahnemann they were not so frank as Von Behring, who publicly acknowledged his indebtedness to Hahnemann for the idea of his diphtheritic antitoxin and declared that no other word than "Homœopathy" would adequately explain its modus operandi.

I have dwelt somewhat upon this subject, not only because it shows Hahnemann's priority and supremacy as an original investigator and thinker, but because we have in this cholera episode a complete illustration of the homœopathic teaching in regard to the nature of disease.

The first proposition is that *disease is not a thing but only a condition of a thing;* that disease is only a changed state of health, a perverted vital action, and not in any sense a material or tangible entity to be seen, handled, or weighed, although it may be measured.

Those who think that have been following me closely, warm in their interest in the identification of the comma bacillus as the cause of cholera, are doubtless puzzling their brains to reconcile that identification and demonstration with the statement that "disease is not a thing but a condition of a thing." Has it not been demonstrated that the bacillus is a tangible thing? Those who think thus have overlooked an important point in my statement, and by so doing have identified the conditioning and the conditioned, which is a violation of the rules of logic.

The foundation is a condition for the house, but it is not the house nor the cause of the house. Much less is the house identical with the foundation. The bacillus is the proximate cause of cholera but it is not cholera, nor the sole cause of cholera. It is only one of several conditions necessary for the production and propagation of cholera, all of which must be considered if we are to form just conclusions about the nature of disease. For instance, there are sanitary conditions to be considered, with all their numerous implications; there are social and moral conditions, including facilities and modes of transportation and inter-communication between nations, communities and individuals to be considered. There are also atmospheric and telluric conditions.

It is to be noted that it was only after many trials by administration of the bacillus-cultures that one individual was found who succumbed to the attack. With him there was a condition of individual susceptibility and that susceptibility was an essential condition for him, as it is in all such cases.

Those who did not observe that point were caught napping as many others have been when dealing with such subjects.

We must discriminate between cause and effect, between power and product, between that which acts and that which is acted upon. We must also learn to realize that the power which acts to cause or produce effects is always invisible. We see the wonders of the realm of dynamics only with the eyes of the mind. We know the existence of force only by its manifestations and phenomena. We know gravity, chemical affinity, electricity, life, mind, health, disease, only by their phenomena. We must not let the phenomena which we perceive with our organs of sensation blind us to the existence of the invisible power which produces them, nor think that the visible is the all of existence. The tumor, the eruption, the ulcer, the pain, or the fever which we see or feel, or the germ or bacillus which the microscope reveals, is not the all of disease. Back of these lies the substantial, all-pervading life principle of the organism, which primarily acts and is acted upon.

Functional or dynamic change always precedes tissue changes. Internal changes take place before external signs appear. We do not see the beginnings of disease. Neither do we see disease itself any more than we see life, mind, or thought; for disease, in the last analysis, is primarily only an altered state of life and mind, manifesting itself in morbid functions and sensations, which may or may not lead to visible tissue changes.

All action is conditional. No force or agent acts unconditionally. Our cholera illustration teaches that no pathogenic microorganism acts unconditionally. No germ or bacillus is the sole or absolute cause of any disease, but only a proximate or exciting cause under certain conditions. Other predisposing, contributing, antecedent causes must exist before the germ becomes operative. Numerous Klebs-Loeffler bacilli may be found in the throats of perfectly healthy people who have been in contact with a diphtheria patient. An examination of the nasal or pharyngeal secretions of any one of us at this moment would probably reveal the presence of numerous pathogenic organisms from the inhaled dust of the street. But we are not thereby endangered beyond the ordinary chances of life, because nature has her own means of protection against all such outside, morbific influences. They are harmless to us in our normal condition because the element of morbid susceptibility to these particular germs is absent in the great majority of individuals. The vital resisting power of the healthy individual is superior to the infecting power of the bacilli or any other form of infecting agent, under ordinary conditions. It has been well said that "the best protection against contagion is good health."

It behooves us, therefore, to understand what Hahnemann means by "the sick" in the first paragraph of the Organon, where he says that the first and sole duty of the physician is to heal the sick; and what he means in the third paragraph where he says that the physician should distinctly understand what is curable in disease.

In paragraph six he tells us that in each individual case we are to observe only what is outwardly discernible through the senses; that this consists of changes in the sensorial condition or health of body and soul revealed to our senses by morbid signs or symptoms and that these morbid signs or symptoms, in their entirety, *represent* the disease in its full extent; that they constitute the true and only conceivable form or picture of the disease.

In paragraph seven he tells us that the disease is *the suffering of the "dynamis"* or the life principle of the organism; that the symptoms by which this suffering is made known constitute not only the sole guide to the choice of the curative remedy, but are in themselves all there is to be removed in effecting the cure. They represent "that which is curable in disease."

In paragraph eight he states the general principle in logic, that when an effect ceases we may conclude that the cause has ceased to act. He says that when every perceptible symptom of disease or suffering of the vital force has been removed, the patient is cured.

Note carefully exactly what he says here. He does not say that when every tangible or visible result of the disease has been removed the patient is cured, but that disease is cured when every perceptible *sign of suffering of the dynamis* has been removed.

The patient whose disease has produced a tumor may be perfectly cured by homœopathic remedies and still have his tumor left, precisely as he may have a scar after the perfect healing of a wound.

The tumor is not the disease, but only the "end product" of the disease, as it were. The tumor is not the object of curative treatment, but the disease which preceded and produced the tumor. The tumor, in the course of successful treatment, may or may not be absorbed and disappear. It depends upon the state of the patient's metabolism.

If the patient's vitality has not been too much exhausted by long illness and faulty living or treatment, and if his powers of metabolism are equal to the task, the tumor, or the effusion, or the infarctus or whatever it may be, will be absorbed, as frequently happens in cases treated by skillful prescribers. I have myself seen this happen many times. But if the contrary is the case the tumor, or other morbid product, constitutes a merely mechanical condition which we may turn over to the surgeon for the exhibition of his manual dexterity and technical skill—after the patient has been cured of his disease.

There is another class of cases where medicine and surgery must go hand in hand because of lack of time; where, from seeing the case too late, mechanical conditions have come to constitute a menace to life. But even here skillful homœopathic prescribing greatly lessens the danger of operating and increases the chances of a happy outcome in the cure of the patient.

The mere removal of the tangible products of disease by mechanical means as in the case of tumors, or of the external visible signs of disease by topical applications as in cases of eruptions and discharges, not only does not cure the disease, but does the patient a positive injury and renders the case inveterate or more difficult to cure. Not infrequently it leads to the death of the patient from metastasis and the complications which result from such treatment. Disease is only *cured* by the internally administered similar medicine, with due regard to the proper auxiliary psychical, hygienic and mechanical treatment.

Disease, then, is primarily a morbid disturbance or disorderly action of the vital force, represented by the totality of the symptoms of the patient. It is a purely dynamical disturbance of the vital powers and functions, which may or may not ultimate in gross tissue changes. The tissue changes are no essential part of the disease, but only the products of the disease, which, as such, are not the object of treatment by medication.

Cure, from the homœopathic point of view, consists in "the speedy, gentle and permanent *restitution of health,* or alleviation and obliteration of disease, in its entire extent, in the shortest, most reliable, and safest manner, according to clearly intelligible reasons" or principles.

To remove some symptoms of disease and palliate others is not to remove or obliterate the disease "in its entire extent," nor permanently restore health. Whether palliation makes for the patient's well-being or not depends upon the circumstances and how it is done. We may palliate symptoms and make the patient more comfortable by the use of well-selected homœopathic remedies, or by a judicious and conservative surgical operation; and that may be all it is possible to do in a particular case. Palliation is permissible and all that is possible sometimes. But there is a right way and wrong way to palliate. The wrong way of palliation often leads to metastasis to more important organs. That is always bad for the patient, because it leads to further complications and suffering. The right kind of palliation *is curative as far as it goes, i. e.,* it is achieved by the application of the curative principle; but in the nature of the case, or exigencies of the situation, cure in the complete sense may be impossible, because the case has passed beyond the curable stage. We must learn to distinguish between incurable disease and disease which has reached the incurable stage. There is no such thing as "incurable disease." All diseases are curable before they have reached a certain stage; and that does not necessarily mean that we must "begin to treat a child three hundred years before it is born," as Dr. Oliver Wendel Holmes humorously but pessimistically said.

"Suppression," or palliation of disease, is the removal of the external symptoms of disease by external, mechanical, chemical or topical treatment; or by means of powerful drugs, given internally in massive doses, which have a direct physiological or toxic effect but no true therapeutic or curative action.

The "suppressed" case always "goes bad." As an example of metastasis frequently observed and verified, take the surgical obliteration of a rectal fistula resulting from an ischio-rectal abscess in a tubercular patient, without having previously submitted the patient to a successful course of curative medical and hygienic treatment. What happens in such a case? The local, visible rectal symptoms are removed, the fistula is gone, but what about the patient? Presently the interior systemic disease which, up to the time of the operation may be said to have been tentatively expressing itself in the rectal lesion, to the temporary relief of the organism and protection of vital organs, now breaks out in the lungs and hastens the patient to an untimely grave. A possibly curable case has been rendered incurable and a patient's life sacrificed because the physician or surgeon has failed to recognize the true indications in the case. The abscess and fistula act as if they were the "vent" or "exhaust" of the disease, affording temporary safety to vital organs. Close the exhaust and an explosion follows.

The practical bearing of the foregoing consideration appears when we come to the treatment of disease. If we regard the external, tangible manifestations as the all of disease and make them the object of treatment, we are likely to lose sight of the logical relation between cause and effect, overlook important etiological factors, invert the natural order and direction of treatment and end by using measures which can result only in failure or in mere palliation instead of cure. Such treatment fails because it is one-sided and superficial. It is not guided by knowledge of the true nature and causes of disease and their relation to its external manifestations.

Almost anyone may learn how to drive an automobile; but without a knowledge of the nature, source and mode of application of its motive power and means of control he is likely to be left helpless by the roadside if anything goes wrong with his motor. Life is the power which runs the human automobile, and he who would run it successfully and be able to adjust and repair it when things go wrong must know the nature and laws of that power.

CHAPTER VII

SUSCEPTIBILITY, REACTION AND IMMUNITY

By susceptibility we mean the general quality or capability of the living organism of receiving impressions; the power to react to stimuli. Susceptibility is one of the fundamental attributes of life. Upon it depends all functioning, all vital processes, physiological and pathological. Digestion, assimilation, nutrition, repair, secretion, excretion, metabolism and katabolism, as well as all disease processes arising from infection or contagion depend upon the power of the organism to react to specific stimuli.

The cure and alleviation of diseases depend upon the same power of the organism to react to the impression of the curative remedy.

When we give a drug to a healthy person for the purpose of making a homœopathic "proving" or test, the train of symptoms which follows represents the reaction of the susceptible organism to the specific irritant or stimulus administered.

When a homœopathically selected medicine is administered to a sick person, the disappearance of the symptoms and restoration of the patient to health represents the reaction of the susceptible organism to the impression of the curative remedy.

The "homœopathic aggravation," or slight intensification of the symptoms which sometimes follows the administration of the curative remedy, is merely the reaction of the organism, previously perhaps inactive or acting improperly because of lowered susceptibility, as it responds to the gently stimulating action of the medicine. As a piece of machinery in which the bearings have become dry or rusty from disuse, creaks and groans when it is again started up into action, so the diseased, congested, sluggish organs of the body sometimes squeak and groan when they begin to respond to the action of the curative remedy. All this, and much more is included in the Hahnemann doctrine of Vitality, under the Newtonian principle of Mutual Action, ("Action and reaction are equal and opposite") restated in medical terms by Hahnemann as *"Similia Similibus Curantur,"* and employed by him as the law of therapeutic medication.

It is understood that action and reaction in the medical and physiological sense takes place only in the living organism, and that it depends upon that fundamental quality and attribute of life which we call susceptibility.

We shall see that the kind and degree of reaction to medicines depends upon *the degree of susceptibility* of the patient, and that the kind and degree of susceptibility, in any particular case or patient, depends largely upon how the case is handled by the physician; for it is in his power to modify susceptibility. Indeed, this power to *modify susceptibility* is the basis of the art of the physician.

If the physician knows how to modify susceptibility in such a way as to satisfy the requirements of the sick organism and bring about a true cure, then is he a physician indeed; *since cure consists simply in satisfying the morbid susceptibility of the organism* and putting an end to the influx of disease-producing causes. To accomplish this he must know that susceptibility implies and includes affinity, attraction, desire, hunger, need; that these all exist and express themselves normally as states and conditions in every living being; but that they may become morbid and perverted and so cause disease, suffering and death. He knows also that susceptibility implies the existence of the wherewithal to satisfy susceptibility; to supply need, hunger, desire, affinity, attraction, and he knows how and where to find the necessary modifying agents.

It is a well-known fact that the living organism is much more susceptible to homogeneous or similar stimuli than to heterogeneous or dissimilar stimuli. Throughout the entire vegetable and animal kingdom we find the law of development and growth to be *like appropriating like.* Organism and organs select elements most similar to their own elements. The same law holds good in excretion, each organ excreting or throwing off elements analogous to those of its own basic structure.

So it is in satisfying the morbid susceptibility which constitutes disease. As hunger demands food, so disease demands medicine. But the demand is always consistent with the universal law.

It is for the symptomatically similar medicine, because that is the only thing that really satisfies the susceptibility.

This morbid susceptibility which constitutes disease may exist toward several different medicines, the degree of susceptibility to each depending upon the degree of symptom similarity; but the highest degree of susceptibility exists toward the *most similar*— the simillimum, or equal. Hence, a given patient may be cured of his disease homœopathically by either of two methods; by giving several more or less similar medicines in succession, or by giving one exactly similar medicine—the simillimum or equal. It depends upon whether he is being treated by a bungler or an expert. The bungler may "zig zag" his patient along through a protracted illness and finally get him well, where an expert would cure him by the straight route with a single remedy in half the time.

The sick organism being so much more susceptible to the similar medicine than the well organism, it follows that the size or quantity of the dose depends also upon the degree of susceptibility of the patient. A dose that would produce no perceptible effect upon a well person may cause a dangerous or distressing aggravation in a sick person, just as a single ray of light will cause excruciating pain in an inflamed retina, which in its healthy condition would welcome the full light of day.

Susceptibility as a state may be increased, diminished or destroyed. Either of these is a morbid state which must be considered therapeutically from the standpoint of the individual patient. Morbid susceptibility may be regarded as a negative or minus condition—a state of lowered resistance. J. J. Garth Wilkinson (Epidemic Man and His Visitations) says:

"One man catches scarlet fever from another man, but catches it because he is *vis minor* to the disease, which to him alone is *vis major*. His neighbor does not catch it; his strength passes it by as no concern of his. It is the first man's foible that is the prime reason of his taking the complaint. He is a vacuum for its pressure. The cause why he succumbed was in him long before the infector appeared. Susceptibility to a disease is sure in the individual or his race to be (come) that disease in time. For the air is full of diseases waiting to be employed.

"Susceptibility in organism, mental or bodily, is equivalent to *state.* State involves the attitude of organizations to internal causes and to external circumstances. It is all the resource of defense or the way of yielding. The taking on of states is the history of human life. Pathology is the account of the taking on of diseased states, or of definite forms of disease, mental or bodily.

"In health we live and act and resist without knowing it. In disease we live but suffer; and know *ourself* in conscious or unconscious exaggeration."

We must also predicate a state of normal susceptibility to remedial as well as toxic agencies, which it is the duty of the physician to conserve and utilize. No agent or procedure should be used as a therapeutic measure which has the power to diminish, break down or destroy the normal susceptibility or reactibility of the organism, because that is one of the most valuable medical assets we possess. Without it all our efforts to cure are in vain. To use agents in such a manner or in such a form or quantity as to diminish, impair or destroy the power of the organism to react to stimuli, is to align ourselves with the forces of death and disintegration. Conservation of the power of the organism to react defensively to a toxin, a contagion or an infection is as important as it is to conserve the power to react constructively to food and drink, or curatively to the homœopathic remedy. It is as normal and necessary for the organism to react pathogenetically to a poison, in proportion to the size and power of the dose, as it is to react physiologically to a good dinner.

The problem is one of adjustment to conditions. The point to be kept in mind is to recognize and conserve normal susceptibility in all our dealings with the sick and to do nothing to impair it. Every remedy or expedient proposed for treatment of the sick should be submitted to this test. Does it respond to the demand of the suffering organism as expressed by similar symptoms? Does it supply the organic need? Does it satisfy the susceptibility without injury or impairment of function? In short, *does it cure?* Unquestionably many remedies, methods and processes more or less popular even to-day, in this ultra-scientific age, do not and cannot conform to this standard.

Many substances are used medically in such form, in such doses, by such methods and upon such principles as to be distinctly depressive or destructive of normal reactivity. They are forced upon or into the suffering organism empirically without regard to nature's laws. So far as their effect upon disease is concerned they are in no wise curative, but only palliative or suppressive and the ultimate result, if it be not death, is to leave the patient in a worse state than he was before. Existing disease symptoms are transformed into the symptoms of an artificial drug disease. The organism is overwhelmed by a more powerful enemy which invades its territory, takes violent possession and sets up its own kingdom.

Such victories over disease are a hollow mockery from the standpoint of a true therapeutics.

We do not have to seek far for illustrative examples:

Professor James Ewing, of Cornell University Medical College, in a lecture upon *Immunity* (1909), called the problem of the endotoxins "The stone wall of Serum Therapy." He said:

"The effort to produce passive immunity against the various infections by means of sera may fail in spite of the destruction of all the bacteria present in the body, by reason of the endotoxins thrown out in the process of bacteriolysis resulting from the serum injections.

"The action of endotoxins of all kinds is similar: there is a reduction of temperature *but an active degeneration of the organs—a status infectiosus.* Thus sterile death is produced where cultures from the organs and tissues show that the bacteria in question have all been destroyed; *but the animal dies.*

"This problem of the endotoxins is at present the stone wall of Serum Therapy."

Prof. Ewing cited the case of a patient who received injections of millions of killed gonococci for gonococcic septicæmia; the temperature came down to normal, but the patient died. He continues: "An animal whose serum is normally bacteriolytic may, on immunization, lose this power; the bacteria *living in the serum, but not producing symptoms.*

"Thus, a rabbit's serum is normally bacteriolytic to the typhoid bacillus, but the rabbit is susceptible to infection. If, however, the rabbit is highly immunized the serum is no longer bactericidal, *the typhoid bacilli living in the serum,* but the animal not being susceptible of infection. The animal dies."

"It seems therefore that the effort must be made in the future to enable *the tissue and the bacteria to live together in peace rather than to produce a state where the serum is destructive to the bacteria.*"

These are strong and significant words from the highest authority on pathology in America.

In the cases cited by Prof. Ewing we see the destruction, partial or complete, of susceptibility—of the normal power of the organism to react to the stimulus of either the sera or the bacilli.

In the case of total destruction of the susceptibility death followed. The condition of the patients in whom destruction was only partial may be better imagined than described. A rabbit or a man, whose fluids and tissues are in such a depraved or vitiated state that typhoid or other virulent organisms live and thrive in them without producing symptoms, and who will no longer react to a powerful serum, is not in a state of health to say the least. It is a condition which reminds us of the scathing words of Jesus;—"Woe unto you, Scribes and Pharisees, hypocrites! for ye are like whited sepulchres, which indeed appear beautiful outwardly, *but within are full of dead men's bones and all uncleanness.*"

The use of *antiseptics* in the treatment of disease, or surgically (in the field of operation), is another means of impairing or destroying normal susceptibility.

Articles have appeared in leading medical journals of the dominant school (Boston Surgical Journal, and the Therapeutic Gazette), in which it was pointed out that the use of antiseptics in the treatment of tonsillitis increased the inflammation, prolonged the disease and retarded convalescence. It was explained that by diminishing the number of bacteria in the crypts which were generating toxin, the period required for the formation of the requisite amount of anti-bodies was unduly prolonged. They had just waked up to the fact that the living organism, even if diseased, has some means of self-protection and that, other things being equal, the automatic formation of the antitoxins and anti-bodies in the organism goes on at about an equal pace with the generation of toxins.

The destructive action of the antiseptics upon the living tissue cells and phagocytic leucocytes of the host—otherwise the patient

—was also pointed out as contraindicating their use by these discerning authorities. In destroying these bodies we are destroying the physical basis of life itself. We slay our best friends. They further showed that the depression of vitality thus caused resulted later in increase of fever and cervical adenitis, due to the increased absorption of toxins. What they failed to see and explain, however, was *that the increased fever and inflammation were in reality the manifestation of that vital reaction or resistance on the part of the organism, which is the means by which the real, natural curative antibodies and antitoxins are produced,* and that this should never be interfered with.

Inflammation and fever are not evils *per se*. They are merely the signs of normal reaction and resistance to an irritant or poison by which nature protects herself. They are not enemies to be resisted, but friends and allies to be co-operated with in the destruction of a common enemy.

Inflammation and fever mean simply greater vital activity, more rapid circulation, respiration and oxygenation, more rapid and thorough elimination of waste or toxic substances, and the concurrent formation of natural antitoxins and antibodies by means of which recovery is brought about.

Pain, inflammation and fever are not the real disease nor the real object of treatment. To view them as such leads logically and inevitably to mere palliation or suppression of symptoms, than which there are no greater medical evils. It is based upon a false and illogical interpretation of the phenomena of disease which mistakes results for causes.

Stimulants and Depressants.—Prof. James C. Wood, veteran surgeon and author of Cleveland, Ohio, in a letter to the writer, dated February 20, 1922, following the publication of this article in the Homœopathic Recorder, wrote as follows:

"There is one remedy you have omitted in your discussion of shock, namely, strychnia or nux vomica. Crile in his experimental work on shock has shown that it is almost impossible to differentiate true shock from strychnia poisoning. As a result of his experimentation surgeons have pretty largely discarded strychnia in the treatment of shock, Crile proving that they are killing more than they are curing by full doses of strychnia in dealing with the same. On the other hand, I am using it in *small doses* with the greatest possible advantage, showing conclusively, I think, its homœopathicity in shock."

It seems to be pretty well established that alcohol, the typical and perhaps most commonly used stimulant, adds nothing to the physiological forces of the body. It takes of what might be called the "reserve fund" of organic force and uses it up a little faster than nature would otherwise permit. It acts like the whip to the tired horse, not like rest, water and food, which nourish, strengthen, repair and replace worn-out tissues. Its action on the brain and nerves is well known. Many have seen, on the dissecting table, the characteristic watery, contracted brain of the chronic alcoholic. We know the power of alcohol to harden and shrivel and devitalize organic tissues. Its power to paralyze the vaso-motor system is seen in the flushed face, congested capillaries and ruby nose of the inebriate. We are aware of its inhibiting effect upon the sensory nerves, by which it makes its victim insensible to the impressions of heat, cold and pain, so that, in extreme intoxication, he falls on a red-hot stove and is burned to death, or staggers into a snow bank and freezes to death without knowing it.

All these things define the nature and measure of power of alcohol to decrease or destroy normal susceptibility.

Less only in proportion to the amount used is its influence to lessen susceptibility when used as a stimulant in disease. Here, as in all other realms, the law holds good: "Action and reaction are equal and opposite." Stimulation and depression are equal and opposite. Whip the exhausted horse and he will go on a little ways and then drop. No amount of whipping will start him up again. He soon reaches a point where his susceptibility to that kind of a stimulant is exhausted. Overstimulate the weakened or exhausted patient and the same thing will happen.

This is not to say that there is no place for physiological drug stimulants in the healing art, but only to point out that the place which they legitimately fill is an exceedingly small one and rarely met. Certain rare cases of typhoid fever, diphtheria, and perhaps a few other similar conditions, may be benefited by very small doses of pure brandy and tided over a crisis by that means when they might otherwise die. But the amount of stimulant necessary to accomplish that end is extremely small. More than the necessary amount will assuredly hasten death, because the margin of strength is so small the least waste by overuse may prove fatal.

The proper use of stimulants in the type of cases referred to was once illustrated by Dr. P. P. Wells. In a critical case of typhoid fever which he saw in consultation, the patient had suffered a severe hemorrhage from the bowels, was very weak, nearly unconscious and had a *soft compressible pulse*. Dr. Wells directed that six drops of brandy be put into six teaspoonfuls of milk and the whole given in three doses of two teaspoonfuls each, at intervals of two hours; to be repeated if reaction did not follow. The effect was surprising. Reaction quickly followed and the patient made a rapid recovery.

We may smile at the size of the dose until we recall how many patients in a similar condition have died under tablespoonful doses of brandy, or hypodermics of strychnia and whiskey. Dr. Wells knew how to correctly measure a patient's susceptibility and he knew how to conserve the last, feeble, flickering remnant of vitality in such cases and make the best of it. He knew better than to waste it by violent measures, as is so often done in cases of shock when hypodermics of brandy and strychnine and other powerful stimulants are used.

The idea held by many that large and powerful doses and strenuous measures are necessary in such cases is entirely wrong. The conception of disease and the interpretation of symptoms is wrong. The resultant treatment is wrong. The imaginary idea of violence, of the malignity and rapidity of *the disease,* is forced to the front and dwelt upon until it seems rational to believe that the treatment must also be violent, active, "heroic." This is practicing homœopathy with a vengeance!

Such an error arises naturally from considering the *disease* to the exclusion of the *patient. Look at the patient* who is suffering from shock. He is pale, his features are sunken, his skin and muscles relaxed, he is covered with a cold, clammy sweat. His respiration is feeble, his pulse almost or quite extinct, he is perhaps almost or quite unconscious. Everything indicates that life and strength are at lowest ebb. The store of vital energy is almost exhausted. The margin left to work upon is very narrow. There is but a step between him and death. The slightest false move, the least violence, is likely to force him across the line which marks the boundary between life and death.

If there is any condition which would seem to demand the use of mild, of the *very* mildest and most delicate, means, this is one. Reaction, as an expression of susceptibility in such cases, is like the love of fair women—something to be wooed delicately; not brutally and fiercely as among barbarians. The condition of shock, or of extreme exhaustion, is no occasion for heroic doses or strenuous measures, but rather for the greatest gentleness and most refined doses. Let the patient inhale camphor, or vinegar, or ammonia (very carefully) if only these domestic remedies are at hand; or give him two or three-drop doses of brandy in a teaspoonful of water; if that is at hand. Teaspoonful doses of hot black coffee may be useful. But as soon as possible, give our potentiated Arnica, Arsenicum, Nux vomica, Veratrum or Carbo veg. or whatever other remedy may be indicated by the etiology and symptoms of the case. The results will be infinitely better than the results of the strenuous method.

"Never," said Dr. Wells, "give brandy or any other stimulant with *a hard and wiry pulse.*"

Deficient reaction or diminished susceptibility may exist in a case or appear during treatment and constitute a condition requiring special treatment. This is especially true in the treatment of chronic diseases, where improvement ceases and well-selected remedies do not seem to act. Under such circumstances it may sometimes be necessary to give a dose of what is called an "intercurrent remedy." Bœnninghausen mentions as appropriate in such cases: Carbo veg., Lauroc., Mosch., Op., Sulph. To these may be added the typical nosodes: Medorr., Psor., Pyrog., Tuberc., Syphil., and also Thuja. The choice of any particular one of these remedies must be governed by the history and symptoms.

Excessive reaction, or irritability, is a condition sometimes met where the patient seems to suffer an aggravation from every remedy, without corresponding improvement. There is a state of general hypersensitiveness.

For such a state, Bœnninghausen recommends Asar., Cham., Coff., China, Ign., Nux v., Puls., Teuc. and Valer.

Aggravation after Mercury requires Hep. or Nit. ac.

Therapeutic suggestion is of use in all such cases, to calm and soothe terrified or excited patients. But in these, as in all other cases, the case and remedy must be carefully individualized.

We see, therefore, that the cure or successful treatment of disease depends not only upon conserving and utilizing the natural susceptibility of the living organism, but on properly adjusting both remedy and dose to the needs of the organism so that susceptibility shall be satisfied, normal reaction induced and equilibrium or health restored. The "Law of the Least Plus" should never be forgotten:—"The quantity of action necessary to effect any change in nature is *the least possible.*"

Immunity which is obtained at the cost of the integrity and purity of the vital organism and its fluids is too dearly purchased.

Inoculation of crude, pathological products like animal sera and vaccines confers only a spurious immunity through impairment or destruction of normal susceptibility. It results in the contamination or poisoning of the entire organism, sets up a morbid condition instead of a healthy one and leads to physical degeneration.

The homœopathic remedy, correctly chosen upon indications afforded by the anamnesis and symptoms of the disease as manifested in the individual and the community, and administered in infinitesimal doses, *per oram,* satisfies the morbid susceptibility, supplies the need of the organism and confers a true immunity by promoting *health,* which is the true object to be gained.

CHAPTER VIII

GENERAL PATHOLOGY OF HOMŒOPATHY

Theory of the Chronic Diseases.—Human pathology is the science which treats of diseased or abnormal conditions of living human beings. It is customary to divide the subject into general pathology and special pathology. *Special pathology* is divided into *medical pathology,* dealing with internal morbid conditions, and *surgical pathology,* which deals with external conditions. *General pathology* bears the same relation to special pathology that philosophy bears to the special sciences. It is the synthesis of the analyses made by special pathology. It deals with principles, theories, explanations and classifications of facts.

While the findings and conclusions of modern pathology are accepted in large part by all schools of medicine, and serve as the common basis of the therapeutic art, there are enough variations and differences, particularly in general pathology, arising from contemplation of the subject from the homœopathic point of view to justify the creation of a special field or department, called Homœopathic General Pathology, especially as it is concerned with *Chronic Diseases.*

Homœopathy differs with regular medicine in its interpretation and application of several fundamental principles of science. It is these differences of interpretation and the practice growing out of them which give homœopathy its individuality and continue its existence as a distinct school of medicine.

These differences are primarily philosophical. They have to do mainly with the interpretation or explanation of facts upon which all are agreed, and which all accept. These differing interpretations arise from differing viewpoints. Modern science in general, and medical science in particular, regards the facts of the universe from a materialistic standpoint. It endeavors to reduce all things to the terms of *matter and motion.* No valid objection could be raised to this if its definitions of these terms were broad enough to include all the facts. But failing in this, and deliberately closing its eyes and refusing to see certain great, fundamental facts which are not covered by its definitions and of which, therefore, no explanation can be made, medical science formulates systems and methods of practice which are not only inefficient, but often positively harmful.

Homœopathic medical science views the facts of the universe in general, and medical facts in particular, from a vitalistic—substantialistic standpoint; that is, from the standpoint of the substantial philosophy, which regards all things and forces, *including life and mind,* as substantial entities, having a real, objective existence. In homœopathic philosophy life and mind are the fundamental verities of the universe.

Upon the recognition of this basic fact rests Hahnemann's doctrine of the "Vital Force" as set forth in the Organon, about which there has been so much discussion. All doubt as to Hahnemann's position is removed and the subject is placed beyond controversy so far as he is concerned by the final sixth revised edition of the Organon, which is at last accessible to the profession. In this edition Hahnemann invariably uses the term, *Vital Principle* instead of Vital Force, even speaking in one place of *"the vital force of the Vital Principle,"* thus making it clear that he holds firmly to the substantialistic view of life—that is, that Life is a substantial, objective entity; a primary, originating power or principle and not a mere condition or mode of motion. From this conception arises the dynamical theory of disease upon which is based the Hahnemann pathology, *viz.:* that disease is always primarily a morbid dynamical or functional disturbance of the vital principle; and upon this is reared the entire edifice of therapeutic medication, governed by the law of *Similia* as a selective principle.

As this view leads to a radically different method of practice, the necessity for a special consideration of general pathology in its various departments is evident.

In formulating his "Theory of the Chronic Miasms," Hahnemann did for pathology what he had already done for therapeutics: he reduced a great mass of unsystematized data to order by making a classification based upon general principles.

This classification of the phenomena of disease led to the

broadest generalization in pathology and etiology that has ever been made, and greatly simplified and elucidated the whole subject.

Hahnemann's generalization was based upon his new and far-reaching discovery: *the existence of living, specific, infectious micro-organisms* as the cause of the greater part of all true diseases.

The history of the progress of natural history shows how men first approached nature; how the facts have been collected, and how these facts have been converted into science by successively broader and broader generalizations leading to the discovery of basic laws of nature.

The work of Hahnemann in pathology may be compared to that of Cuvier in zoology, who reduced the entire animal kingdom to four fundamental classes, based upon the general characteristics of their internal structure: Vertebrates, Mollusks, Articulates and Radiates. Until Cuvier's time there was no great principle of classification. Facts were accumulated and more or less systematized, but they were not arranged according to law.

Hahnemann reduced all the phenomena of chronic disease according to their causes to four fundamental classes, Occupational or drug diseases, Psora, Syphilis and Sycosis.

Taking the entire mass of morbid phenomena, he first eliminated all of the numerous symptoms and so-called diseases which are merely local, temporary and functional, in persons otherwise healthy, due to non-specific causes, such as indiscretions in diet or regimen, mechanical injuries, undue exertions or indulgences, emotional excesses, etc. Such conditions are not true diseases, but mere indispositions, which disappear of themselves under ordinary circumstances when the cause is removed, or yield easily to corrective hygienic, dietetic, moral or mechanical measures. They ordinarily require no medicine. In this class of cases are included many of the so-called occupational diseases, caused by exposure of healthy persons to noxious influences incidental to environment or vocation, such as unsanitary dwellings, exposure to fumes and emanations from chemicals, absorption of minerals such as lead or copper, etc.

The treatment of such conditions involves merely the removal of the cause, and, in some cases, antidoting the poisons, chemically or dynamically.

This removed a large part of the mass of phenomena from the category of diseases and cleared the way for further new classification of the remainder.

The next step consisted in collecting into a class all the phenomena known to be due to those ancient, widespread and malignant scourges of mankind, the venereal diseases. Syphilis, already recognized as the fundamental cause of a large number of symptoms and as a complicating factor in many diseases, had been studied quite extensively. A careful review and collection of all the known phenomena of syphilis was made, greatly enlarging its scope.

Gonorrhœa as a constitutional disease was but little known, but Hahnemann's keen mind had detected its relation to many evil consequences following the suppression of the primary discharge by local treatment. He had also observed the evils arising from the topical and mechanical treatment of the anomalous venereal condition variously known as *Sycosis,* or the "fig wart disease," condylomata, ficus marisca, atrices and warts. (London Medical Dictionary, 1819.)

Certain forms of condylomata were regarded by some authorities as due to syphilis. Although it was known that the tumors were sometimes of venereal origin and accompanied by a kind of gonorrhœal discharge from the genital passages or the rectum, they were not recognized as the manifestations of a distinct disease, differing in many important respects from syphilis, nor were they necessarily connected with gonorrhœa.

Condylomata were not regarded as having any connection with the large number of peculiar constitutional symptoms which are present in many cases. Hahnemann made extensive researches in the phenomena presenting in such cases and came to the conclusion, first, that they constituted a definite and distinct infectious, constitutional venereal disease, clearly distinguishable from syphilis on the one hand, and the simple, non-specific urethritis on the other; and second, that it was due to the presence of specific, living micro-organisms.

To this newly recognized pathological form he applied the generic name *Sycosis,* using the Greek term commonly employed in his day to designate the typical physical manifestation, the "fig wart." His researches in the general subject of syphilis and gonorrhœa, conducted by the inductive method in science, resulted in throwing a flood of light upon a previously obscure subject, more clearly defining and greatly broadening not only the sphere of the venereal diseases, but the scope of all subsequent research. He was thus the precursor by more than fifty years of Noeggerath, who called attention anew to the importance of gonorrhœa as a constitutional disease and demonstrated the gonococcus as its specific proximate cause.

There still remained the vast number of symptoms constituting the non-venereal diseases, acute and chronic, which afflict mankind. These for the most part had been or were being classified in the most arbitrary and whimsical manner.

Classifications and nomenclature were being changed constantly according to the varying opinions and theories of individuals, none of whom were guided by any general principle. The situation was exactly like that which confronted Cuvier in natural history and Linnæus in botany.

Into this wilderness of conflicting names, theories and classifications Hahnemann began to blaze his way, guided by the compass of logic encased in the inductive method of Bacon. His search was now directed to the discovery of the fundamental causes of the non-venereal diseases. Having found that so large a number of symptoms and diseases had a venereal origin in syphilis and sycosis, it occurred to him that it might be possible to find a common, general or primary cause for all, or at least a great part of the remaining symptoms of disease, and thus to make a final generalization. To this end he directed his efforts. Rejecting existing classifications; searching, collecting, comparing, grouping similar and naturally related symptoms in the light of history, logic and experience; tracing the relations between similar diseases and their antecedents, and tracing recognized proximate causes to their antecedent causes as far back as possible, he gradually narrowed the field of general causation until he arrived at one primary cause, which accounted for and explained the greater part, if not all of the phenomena with which he was working.

The determination of a primary cause opened the way for a consistent reclassification of the secondary causes, and the correction of many errors of grouping and nomenclature of diseases. It obliterated at one stroke a large number of fictitious diseases which were in reality named from merely single symptoms. (Hydrocephalus, fever, diarrhœa, hydrophobia, jaundice, diabetes, anæmia, chlorosis, pyorrhœa, otorrhœa, catarrh, eczema, etc., all of which belong to the general class of infections.)

As Cuvier's work showed that the animal kingdom was built on four different structural plans, so, by singular coincidence, Hahnemann's work showed that diseases were built, as it were, on four different plans, according as they arose from four different causes; namely, Occupational or Drug diseases, Syphilis, Sycosis and Psora.

Relation of Bacteriology to Homœopathy.—This brings us to a consideration of Hahnemann's epoch-making discovery of specific, living micro-organisms as the cause of infectious diseases such as cholera and the venereal diseases, and of the relation of bacteriology to homœopathy.

The great practical value of Hahnemann's Theory of the Chronic Diseases has never been fully appreciated because it has never been fully understood.

Hahnemann was so far ahead of his time that his teaching, in its higher phases, could not be fully understood until science in its slower advance had elucidated and corroborated the facts upon which he based it; and this science has done in a remarkable manner. For the suggestion of bacteriology as the basis of a rational modern interpretation of Hahnemann's Theory of the Chronic Diseases we are indebted to the late Dr. Thomas G. McConkey, of San Francisco. His paper, "Psora, Sycosis and Syphilis," published in the December, 1908, number of *The North American Journal of Homœopathy*, laid the profession under a deep obligation to him. The critical insight, originality, open-mindedness and evident comprehension of the deep significance of the facts of the case displayed in that brief but suggestive paper add poignancy to our regrets that he did not live to work out a fuller exposition of the subject himself.

It is perhaps less important that Hahnemann should be accorded the just recognition due him for his remarkable contribution to medical science, than that the world should be given the benefit of the practical teaching included in his Theory of the Chronic Diseases.

Modern bacteriological science, by long independent research, slowly arrived at the goal Hahnemann reached more than half a century before in regard to the nature and causes of certain forms of disease. It has accomplished much in the way of prophylaxis, sanitation and hygiene through the use of that knowledge; but the profession at large has failed to follow his logical and practical deductions in regard to the *cure of these diseases,* or to discover a means of cure for itself. In this respect modern medicine is no further advanced that it was in Hahnemann's day. It is obliged to confess and does confess, when driven to the wall, that it has no reliable cure for any disease.

Vaccine treatment, for example, the latest, most general and most widely adopted theory and practice growing out of bacteriology is now acknowledged by the highest representative authority of regular medicine to be a failure.

The *Journal of the American Medical Association* (No. 21, 1916), presents, as the leading article of that issue, a paper by Dr. Ludwig Hektoen, on "Vaccine Treatment," and devotes to it a page of editorial comment.

The editorial opens as follows:

"Looking backward over the development of active immunization by vaccines during the last fifteen years, we appear to be at the termination of one epoch in the therapeutics of infectious disease. In this issue Hektoen traces the stages by which vaccines which were first employed with attempted scientific control have come into indiscriminate and unrestrained use, with no guide beyond the statements which commercial vaccine makers are pleased to furnish with their wares. Already most physicians are realizing that the many claims made for vaccines are not borne out by facts, and that judging from practical results there is something fundamentally wrong with the method as at present so widely practiced. As clearly shown by Hektoen, 'the simple fact is that we have no reliable evidence to show that vaccines, as used commonly, have the uniformly prompt and specific curative effects proclaimed by optimistic enthusiasts and especially by certain vaccine makers, who manifestly have not been safe guides to the principles of successful and rational therapeutics.'"

It is not fair, and certainly not ingenuous, as that keen critic,

Dr. E. P. Anshutz, then editor of *The Homœopathic Recorder,* pointed out, to put the blame for this failure upon the manufacturer, since *"Vaccine therapy was born in the innermost chamber of laboratory science."*

The editorial concludes as follows:

"The fact that much time and effort of the past ten years appear now to have been wasted, so far as positive results go, should make us doubly cautious in accepting a new and somewhat similar procedure until opportunity has been afforded for its verification under conditions favorable for scientific control."

Confronted with demonstrations of cure by homœopathic medication in such bacterial diseases as cholera, typhoid, typhus and yellow fever, croup, diphtheria, pneumonia, rheumatism and even tuberculosis and cancer, the dominant school of medicine has thus far declined to consider them, denied both the cures and the principles upon which they are accomplished, and continued to follow its traditional course. It still pursues the ancient "will o' the wisp" "specifics for diseases," ever failing and refusing to see that cure is always *individual,* in the *concrete case or patient,* never in the generalized disease; and that such a thing as a specific cure for a disease does not, and, in the nature of things, cannot exist, since no two cases, even of the same disease, are ever the same. Realization of such failures, and bacteriological confirmation of the teaching of Hahnemann in respect to the nature and cause of certain diseases, taken together, should at least create a presumption in favor of the truth of his teaching in regard to the cure of those diseases and lead to a scientific investigation of his method.

Dr. McConkey, viewing Hahnemann's theory from the standpoint of bacteriology, pointed out, first, that we have inherited from preceding generations a false and misleading interpretation of what Hahnemann really taught in regard to *Psora* as the cause of chronic non-venereal diseases.

The primary error consisted in regarding psora merely as a *dyscrasia* or diathesis, which is directly opposed to what Hahnemann taught as we now understand it. Instead of regarding psora as a dyscrasia Hahnemann *included several of the dycrasiæ* among the morbid conditions and diseases *caused by psora.*

Such an error could only have arisen in minds already prejudiced by the current erroneous teaching of the day, and not yet enlightened by knowledge which was soon to come as a result of original research in the field of bacteriology. On this ground it is conceivable how the error arose and spread. New truth, quickly grasped by a few alert and open minds, penetrates the average mind slowly. Original investigators themselves, absorbed in their own pursuit, are often reluctant to consider their work in its relation to the work of preceding investigators, even if they are philosophically competent to do so, which, as a rule, they are not.

The exceptional work of an individual forerunner, therefore, may easily be overlooked for a time; but eventually the truth discovered by him will be recognized, as it now has been in the case of Hahnemann.

Hahnemann was the first to perceive and teach the *parasitical nature* of infectious or contagious diseases, including syphilis, gonorrhœa, leprosy, tuberculosis, cholera, typhus and typhoid fevers; and the *chronic diseases in general,* other than occupational diseases and those produced by drugs and unhygienic living, the so-called drug diseases.

Hahnemann held that all chronic diseases are derived from *three primary, infectious, parasitic sources*. "All chronic diseases," he says, "show such a constancy and perseverance * * * as soon as they have developed and have not been healed by the medical art, that they evermore increase with the years and during the whole of man's lifetime; and they cannot be diminished by the strength (resistance) belonging even to the most robust constitutions. Still less can they be overcome and extinguished. Thus they never pass away by themselves, but increase and are aggravated even until death. They must therefore have for their origin and foundation *constant chronic miasms,* whereby their *parasitical existence* in the human organism is enabled to continually *rise* and *grow*." *(Only living beings grow.)*

A misunderstanding of the sense in which Hahnemann uses the word "miasm" has deceived many. It was the word loosely used in his time to express the morbific emanations from putrescent organic matter, animal or vegetable, and sometimes the effluvia arising from the bodies of those affected by certain diseases, some of which were regarded as infectious and others not.

A misleading distinction was also made between miasma and contagion and between contagion and infection.

Parr's Medical Dictionary, London, 1819, now a very rare book, but the highest authority of that time, article, "Miasma," says: "In the more strict pathological investigation of modern authors they are distinguished from contagion, which is confined to the effluvia from the human body, when subject to disease; yet the contagion, when it does not proceed immediately from the body, but has been for some time confined in clothes, is sometimes styled *miasma*. Another kind of miasma (see contagion) is putrid vegetable matter, and indeed everything of this kind which appears *in the form of air*. Miasma, then, strictly speaking, *is an aerial fluid, combined with atmospheric air,* and not dangerous unless the air be loaded with it. * * *

"Each infectious disease has its own variety, *diffused around the person which it has attacked*, and liable to convey the disease at different distances, according to the nature of the complaint, or to the predisposition of the object exposed to it."

Under "Contagion or Infection" the same authority says: "It has been lately attempted to distinguish these two words, though not with a happy discrimination. We should approach more nearly to common language if we employed the adjective 'infectious' to *disease communicated by contact;* for we *infect* a lancet and we catch a fever by *contagion*. * * * Contagion then exists *in the atmosphere,* and we know distinctly but one kind, *viz.:* Marsh-miasmata, which probably consists of *inflammable air*."

The yellow fever of America, epidemic catarrhs, plague, dysentery, scarlatina, Egyptian ophthalmia, jail, hospital and other fevers, smallpox, measles, ulcerated throat, whooping cough, the itch, venereal diseases and the yaws, are mentioned as examples of miasmatic diseases, some of which are regarded as "infectious," and others not. "Other complaints supposed to be infectious are apparently so from their being the offspring of *contagion* (that is, 'aerial fluids, combined with atmospheric air') only."

."People are very variously susceptible to infection. The slightest breath will sometimes induce the disease, while others will daily breathe the poisonous atmosphere without injury."

GENERAL PATHOLOGY OF HOMŒOPATHY 97

"Infection is indeed more often taken than is supported. * * * It is generally·*received with the air in breathing.*"

This shows the confused state of medical opinion at the time when Hahnemann was conducting his investigations of the subject, which were to result in his propounding the most startling, revolutionary and far-reaching theory in the history of medicine, namely, the *parasitical nature of infectious and chronic diseases.*

That Hahnemann, in using the word *miasm,* had something more in mind than "an aerial fluid mixed with atmospheric air," is proven not only by his use of the word "parasitical," but by his several references to the *"living beings"* of which his "miasma" were composed.

In a strong protest (1830), against the current, terribly pernicious atmospheric-telluric theory of the nature of cholera Hahnemann stated the infectious, miasmatic-parasitic nature of cholera and described its rise and growth in the following words: "The most striking examples of infection and rapid spread of cholera take place * * * in this way: On board ships in those confined spaces, filled with mouldy, watery vapors, the cholera miasm finds a favorable element for its multiplication, and *grows* into an enormously increased *brood* of those excessively *minute, invisible, living creatures,* so inimical to human life, of which the *contagious matter* of the cholera most probably consists."

"* * * This concentrated aggravated miasm kills several members of the crew. The others, however, being frequently exposed to the danger of infection and thus gradually habituated to it, at length become fortified against it (immunized) and no longer liable to be infected. These individuals, apparently in good health, go ashore and are received by the inhabitants without hesitation into their cottages, and ere they have time to give an account of those who have died of the pestilence on board the ship, those who have approached nearest to them are suddenly carried off by the cholera. The cause of this is undoubtedly the invisible cloud that hovers closely around the sailors who have remained free from the disease, composed of probably millions of those miasmatic *animated beings,* which, at first developed on the broad, marshy bank of the tepid Ganges, always searching out in preference the human being to his destruction and attaching themselves closely to him, when transferred to distant and even colder regions, become habituated to these also, without any diminution either of their unhappy *fertility* or of their fatal destructiveness."

"This pestiferous, infectious *matter,*" he calls it, " which is *carried* about in the clothes, hair, beard, soiled hands, instruments, etc., of physicians, nurses and others," seems to spread the infection and cause epidemics.

Here we have an anticipation by more than fifty years of Koch's discovery of the comma bacilli of cholera. The names, bacilli, bacteria, microbes, micro-organisms, etc., had not been invented in Hahnemann's time, nor had the microscope, with which Koch was able to verify the truth of Hahnemann's idea, been invented. Hahnemann had no microscope, but he had a keen, analytical mind, phenomenal intuition, logic and reasoning powers, and vast erudition. He used the terminology of his day, which he qualified to suit his purpose and thus made it clear that by the word "miasma," amplified by the descriptive terms "Infectious, contagious, excessively minute, invisible *living creatures"* as applied to cholera, he meant precisely what we mean today when we use the terms of bacteriology to express the same idea.

Hahnemann's elaborate and exhaustive studies of the nature and causes of chronic diseases had previously paved the way for his theory of the nature of cholera. In these studies he extended and applied the principle of *Anamnesis* to the critical study of a large number of cases of many different diseases.

First analyzing these diseases into their symptomatic elements, he proceeded to make a new three-fold classification:

"If we accept those diseases which have been created by a perverse medical practice, or by deleterious labors in quicksilver, lead, arsenic, etc. (occupational diseases) which appear in the common pathology under a hundred proper names as supposedly separate and well-defined diseases (and also those springing from *syphilis,* and the still rarer ones springing from *sycosis*), *all the remaining natural chronic diseases, whether with names or without them, find in Psora their real origin, their only source,"*

We have thus:
1. Drug and occupational diseases.

2. Infectious venereal diseases.
3. All other natural chronic diseases.

Excluding Classes 1 and 2, he found that all the diseases in Class 3 were related, directly or indirectly, and could be traced to *one primary cause.*

After many years of patient historical and clinical investigation he found that cause to be an ancient, almost universally diffused, contagious or infectious principle embodied in *a living parasitical, micro-organism,* with an incredible capacity for multiplication and growth. This organism and the disease produced by it he named *Psora* (Gr. *Psora*-itch). He did not invent the name but chose it, first, because he found that originally, the disease manifested itself mostly on the skin and external parts; and second, because the cutaneous manifestations of the diseases which spring from this cause were accompanied, in their original form, by intense itching and burning.

In all such diseases the contagion is conveyed by contact. Research showed that the great fundamental disease thus identified and named, is the oldest, most universal, most pernicious and most misapprehended chronic parasitic disease in existence. "For thousands of years," Hahnemann says, "it has disfigured and tortured mankind; and, during the last centuries, it has become the cause of those thousands of incredibly different, acute as well as chronic non-venereal diseases with which the civilized portion of mankind becomes more and more infected upon the whole inhabited globe."

Hahnemann estimated that seven-eighths of the chronic diseases of his day were due to psora, the remaining eighth being due to syphilis and sycosis.

The Doctrine of Latency.—Hahnemann taught that psora, like syphilis and sycosis, may remain latent for long periods, "until circumstances awaken the disease slumbering within and thus develop *its germs."* This doctrine of latency was strenuously opposed for a long time, but is now endorsed and taught by the highest authorities in regard to syphilis, gonorrhœa and tuberculosis.

Behring and other authorities on tuberculosis now hold that the infection often occurs in infancy or young life and remains latent until later life. Hahnemann's doctrine of latency is therefore confirmed by modern research in regard to tuberculosis, as it has long been of syphilis, and, for a shorter period, of gonorrhœa.

"The oldest monuments of history," says Hahnemann, "show the *Psora* even then in great development. Moses, 3400 years ago pointed out several varieties. In Leviticus, chapter 13, and chapter 21, verse 20, where he speaks of the bodily defects which must not be found in a priest who is to offer sacrifice, malignant itch is designated by the word *Garab,* which the Alexandrian translators (In the Septuagint) translated with *psora agria,* but the Vulgate with *Scabies jugis.* The Talmudic interpreter, Johnathan, explained it as *dry itch spread over the body;* while the expression, *Yalephed,* is used by Moses for *lichen, tetter, herpes.* (See M. Rosenmueller, *Scholia in Levit.,* p. 11, edit. sec., p. 124.)

The commentators in the so-called English Bible-work also agree with this definition, Calmet among others saying: "Leprosy is similar to an inveterate itch with violent itching." The ancients also mention the peculiar, characteristic, *voluptuous* itching which attended itch then as now, while after the scratching a painful burning follows: among others Plato, who calls itch *glykypikron,* while Cicero remarks the *dulcedo* of *scabies."*

"At that time (Moses) and later on among the Israelites, the disease seems to have mostly kept the external parts of the body for its chief seat. This was also true of the malady as it prevailed in uncultivated Greece, later in Arabia, and, lastly, in Europe during the Middle Ages. * * * The nature of this miasmatic itching eruption *always remained essentially the same."*

It is identical, therefore, with the ancient form of leprosy; with the "St. Anthony's Fire," or malignant erysipelas which prevailed in Europe for several centuries and then reassumed the form of leprosy, through the leprosy which was brought back by the returning crusaders in the thirteenth century. After that it spread more than ever. It was gradually modified by greater personal cleanliness, more suitable clothing and general improvement in hygienic conditions, until it was reduced to a "common itch," which could be and was more easily removed from the skin by external treatment.

But Hahnemann points out that the state of mankind was not improved thereby.

In some respects he says, it grew far worse; for although in ancient times the skin disease was very troublesome to its victims, the rest of the body enjoyed a fair share of general health. Moreover, the disgusting appearance of the lepers caused them to be more dreaded and avoided, and their segregation in colonies limited the spread of the infection. This element of safety was lost when the disease assumed its milder appearing form, as the itch, without losing in the slightest degree its infectious-contagious character. The infectious fluid resulting from the scratching, contaminated everything it touched and spread the disease broadcast.

Metastasis.—Many superficial critics have ridiculed the idea that the *itch,* known even before Hahnemann's day to be due to a minute but visible animal parasite, the *acarus scabiei,* was the cause of any other than a local disease of the skin. They did not consider that even if this were true, it might be the host or carrier of another, smaller, infectious micro-organism, in the same way as the flea and the mosquito are carriers of infection. Witty Dean Swift (1667-1745) could have taught them better:

"So naturalists observe, a flea
Has smaller fleas that on him prey,
And these have smaller still to bite 'em,
And so proceed *ad infinitum."*

"Psora has thus become the most infectious and most general of all the chronic miasms," says Hahnemann. The disease, by metastasis from the skin, caused by external palliative treatment, attacks internal organs and causes a multitude of chronic diseases the cause of which is generally unrecognized.

Many have been skeptical of the danger of metastasis of chronic external or skin diseases and this skepticism has led to dire results. It would seem that a physician who dreads and fully realizes the danger of a "repercussion" or metastasis of the eruption of *acute* measles or scarlet fever, with its well-known serious and often fatal consequences in the brain, kidneys or lungs, could not consistently doubt the possibility of the same kind of results from the metastasis of a *chronic* eruption.

Innumerable facts, observed by competent physicians for centuries past, and confirmed in many cases by modern research, make such a position untenable. Metastasis of disease is today an accepted fact in medical science.

Our knowledge of metastasis rests, scientifically, upon our knowledge of *embolism*. "Embolism," says the "American Textbook of Pathology," "rests essentially upon the anatomic and experimental investigation and teachings of Virchow." "Embolism," says this authority, "is the impaction in some part of the vascular system of any undissolved material brought there by the blood current. The material transported in this method is an embolus."

Metastasis is the transference of disease from one part to another not directly connected with it.

Of the several kinds of emboli the "Textbook of Pathology" mentions: "2. Tumor-cells. Emboli composed of *living cells*, capable of farther proliferation, occur in connection with malignant tumors. In carcinoma and sarcoma isolated tumor cells or cell groups, may reach the blood current either indirectly through the lymphatics or directly when the tumor in its growth penetrates the wall and projects into the lumen of a blood vessel. On lodgment the cells proliferate and give rise to secondary tumors. 3. Animal and vegetable parasites. *Bacteria of various kinds,* as well as protozoa and the embryos of a few large animal parasites may be transported by the circulation and act as emboli."

Hahnemann's teaching is thus elucidated and confirmed by pathology. The infectious, parasitic, primary and typical micro-organism of Psora, driven from the skin by local treatment, finds a ready route to deeper tissues, structures and organs through the capillaries, the lymphatic and glandular systems and the nervous system. Here it develops its secondary specific form and character according to its location and the predisposition and environment of the individual, giving rise to a vast number of secondary symptoms.

"So great a flood of numberless nervous symptoms, painful ailments, spasms, ulcers, *cancers,* adventitious formations, *dyscrasias, paralyses, consumptions* and cripplings of soul, mind and body were never seen in ancient times when the Psora mostly confined itself to its dreadful cutaneous symptoms, leprosy.

"Only during the last few centuries has mankind been flooded with these infirmities, owing to the causes first mentioned" (Hahnemann, Chronic Diseases).

The Identity of Psora and Tuberculosis.—Hahnemann

mentions *"consumption, tubercular phthisis,* continual or spasmodic asthma, pleurisy with and without collections of pus in the chest, hemoptysis and suffocative bronchitis," among the known tubercular chest and lung diseases as *due to psora.* He also mentions hydrocephalus, cerebral and cerebro-spinal meningitis, ophthalmia, cataract, tonsilitis, cervical adenitis, otitis, gastric, duodenal and intestinal ulcers; diabetes and nephritis; rachitis and marasmus of children; epilepsy, apoplexy and paralysis; bone and joint diseases; fistulæ; caries and curvature of the spine; encysted tumors; goitre, varices, aneurisms, erysipelas; sarcoma, osteo-sarcoma, schirrus and epithelioma and other diseases, some of which are now known and other of which are thought to be of tubercular origin.

As practically all the diseases known to be due to the tubercle-bacillus are attributed by Hahnemann to Psora, it follows that the cause is identical, *and that the two terms, psora and tuberculosis are synonymous.*

The modern list is growing slowly by additions, from time to time, of other diseases found to be pathologically or bacteriologically related to tuberculosis. It is quite possible that a large part, if not all, of the remainder of Hahnemann's list may ultimately be included in the modern list.

Osler, speaking representatively and with the highest modern authority, agrees with Hahnemann, when he says: *Tuberculosis is the most universal scourge of the human race."*

Hahnemann chose Leprosy as the typical form of the ancient protean disease which he named Psora.

Modern bacteriology finds that the bacilli of leprosy resemble the tubercle bacilli in form, size and staining reactions, and that *the leper reacts to the tuberculin test.*

Saboraud said: *Leprosy is a tubercular disease closely allied to tuberculosis."*

The same staining characteristics are shown by the bacillus smegmatis, the grass and dung bacilli of Mœller, the butter, bacillus of Rabinowitsch and the bacilli from the crypts of the tonsils, described by Marzinowsky.

McConkey, through clinical experience, came to believe and taught that heart disease, with or without valvular lesions, diabetes, rheumatism and cancer were tubercular in nature and origin.

Allen (H. C.) taught the same of typhoid fever. The list might be extended indefinitely.

The writer believes, tentatively, that Acute Anterior Poliomyelitis, etiologically puzzling in spite of the discovery by Flexner of its specific micro-organism, is of tubercular nature and origin.

In considering tuberculosis or psora as a fundamental disease giving rise to many secondary forms of disease, the specific action of the tubercle bacillus must be considered as conditional. No specific organism acts unconditionally. All living germs that propagate and multiply, must have favorable conditions and a suitable soil in which to grow.

Other pathogenic micro-organisms besides the tubercle bacillus, notably the ordinary pyogenic organisms, play their part in the causation and maintenance of the tubercular process. The pyogenic organisms may originate in the teeth, mouth, pharynx, tonsils, nose, ears, or even in the lungs themselves; in the skin, joints, bones, or in short, in almost any organ or tissue of the body where septic processes or lesions exist. But wherever they originate, they play their part in modifying and conditioning the activity of the specific cause of tuberculosis, the bacillus of Koch, and in giving the case its individual character.

Individualization is the cardinal principle of a true pathology as well as of a true therapeutics.

In the eager quest for the specific bacterial causes of the various diseases the principles of logic have not always been applied, and particularly that principle known as the Law of Causation, which teaches that every effect has *a number of causes,* of which the specific cause is only the proximate or most nearly related in the preceding series. It also teaches that the specific cause may be modified in its action on the subject by collateral causes or conditions affecting both the subject and the antecedent causes, so that no specific cause can be said to act unconditionally.

Applying this principle to the subject of individual disease we find that, while specific micro-organisms are a necessary factor as immediate or proximate causes of the respective diseases attributed to them, they only act conditionally, and that many modifying conditions must be considered in assigning them their true relation to individual, concrete cases of disease. It follows that micro-organisms, as causes of individual disease, have a very different kind of importance from that which is commonly assigned to them. They are reduced in rank to an equality with several other related, accessory, contributing causes. The tubercle bacillus, for example, ranks in the individual only equally with constitution, heredity, predisposition and environment. Environment includes social and economic position or condition of life as regards means of subsistence, food, clothing, light, air, housing, neighbors, occupation, mental and physical conditions and habits of life and thought. To conduct a campaign against tuberculosis by directing the efforts principally against the bacilli, while neglecting the numerous other equally important causative factors, is futile and hopeless.

Different also is the kind of importance to be attached to the micro-organism from a therapeutic standpoint. Bacteriology can never serve as a basis for a reliable and efficient therapeutics for the individual. Since the micro-organism is only one of the many causes of disease, the curative remedy for the concrete, resulting disease in the individual must correspond to the combined effects of the various causes. The combined effects are manifested by groups of phenomena or symptoms which vary, more or less, in the various individuals, according to their conditions and circumstances. As the individual cases of every disease vary in their causes and conditions, and consequently in their symptoms or effects, there can be no specific, general remedy for a disease.

It is at this point that the necessity appears for a *general principle of therapeutics*. What is needed is not a general *remedy* for the disease, so long vainly sought, but a general *principle*, applicable to all the varying cases so that the particular remedy needed by each individual may be found. The homœopathic system of therapeutic medication is based upon such a principle, and in that system, combined with rational, moral, hygienic, sanitary and sociological measures is found the solution of the problem.

The Toxicological Theory of Disease.—Life, as a state of existence, has been defined as "a continuous adjustment of internal to external relations."

Every living organism is constantly exposed, at every stage of its existence, to influences from without. The known facts all tend to show that every manifestation of energy on the part of the organism is a reaction to some external agent or influence; or, as it might be put, life, as a state of existence, is the result of constant interaction between the living substance of the organism and the elements of the external world; between the individual and his environment; between the microcosm and the macrocosm.

The specific, exciting or efficient causes of disease are all actually or relatively external to the organism. When a pathogenic agent gains entrance to the living organism, resistance is encountered, a reaction is excited, and the phenomena of that reaction representatively constitute disease. Disease, therefore, is the vital reaction of the living organism to the influence of an agent which is inimical to its welfare. In other words, disease is primarily a *morbid dynamical disturbance* of the vital principle or power which animates the organism, caused by the influence of some morbific agent external to the organism and manifesting itself by perceptible, sensorial, functional and organic symptoms.

It is not sufficient to say, merely, that "disease is a morbid dynamical disturbance of the vital force." That definition is correct as far as it goes, but it stops in the middle. To complete it we must add: "caused by some morbific agent actually or relatively external to the organism;" for every internal effect must have an external cause, and *vice versa*, according to the universal law of cause and effect. From this point of view all diseases may be regarded as intoxications.

All drugs act by virtue of their specific toxic properties.

All bacterial diseases are primarily intoxications or toxæmias.

Pathologists agree that all pathogenic micro-organisms produce their effects in the living body by means of the specific poisons which they secrete while living, or generate after death.

Diseases arising from physical injury or mechanical violence are toxæmias resulting from chemical changes in the injured tissues, brought about by mechanical interference with the circulation and innervation through inhibition of normal functioning, which leads to degenerative changes and the formation of toxins. Localized circulatory stasis, imperfect oxygenation and the inhibitory influence of traumatic shock upon the normal functions and secretions explain the chemico-toxic changes which occur under such conditions.

Disease arising from chemical agents, aside from the direct physical injury or destruction of tissue as by corrosive poisons, are poisonings of the organism.

Disease resulting from mental or physical trauma occur as a result of the toxic chemical or physical changes that take place in the fluids and tissues of the body through the medium of the nervous system, which reacts to the morbid impression of a violent or long-continued mental emotion in the same way that it reacts to any other dynamical disturbance.

If all diseases are the result of some form or degree of poisoning, then in the last analysis *all curative treatment is antidotal treatment,* and cure is accomplished by the use of agents which have the power to antidote or neutralize the poisons and remove their effects.

Physiologically, therapeutically and chemically neutralization is essentially an assimilation.

Since all poisons act pathogenetically on the living organism primarily by virtue of their specific dynamical qualities (as distinguished from their physical and chemical qualities), it follows that the law governing the action of antidotes, if there be such a law, must be a dynamical law. The law of cure appears to be a form or phase of the law of assimilation or reciprocal action, which is dependent upon the law of attraction.

Cure, in the strict sense of the word, can only be accomplished by the use of agents which have the power to neutralize the poisons causing the disease and remove their effects. In other words, all true antidotes, in the medical sense, are physiological or dynamical antidotes, which act specifically according to the physiological or dynamical law of assimilation.

Regular medicine knows no such agents or laws and denies that they exist. From its point of view physiological antidotes are merely: "remedies employed to *combat the symptoms or after effects,* and to neutralize the effects of poisons after absorption into the system. As their name implies, they *do not act on the poison themselves chemically, mechanically, or otherwise, and they are not in this sense true antidotes."* (Ref. Handbook of the Medical Sciences.)

Upon this point hinges the whole controversy between homœopathy and allopathy.

Homœopathy is based, essentially, upon the law of antidotes, which is found by observation, experiment and clinical demonstration to be the law of mutual action or attraction, expressing the equality and contrariety of action and reaction, as manifested in the living organism by similarity of symptoms, and resulting in physiological and chemical assimilation or neutralization.

Antidotes are commonly divided into three classes, according to their mode of action: 1. Physiological or dynamical; 2, chemical, and 3, mechanical.

Dynamical antidotes, in their crude state, are themselves poisons of varying degrees of power. An antidote, in the physiological or dynamical sense, is a toxic substance which, by virtue of its dynamical affinity for another toxic substance, has the power to neutralize that substance and remove its effects. This constitutes cure, the only true antidoting, the working principle of which is applicable in the treatment and cure of diseases as well as of poisonings.

Physiological or dynamical antidoting requires that the antidotal substance shall be pathogenically similar to the poison, but opposite in the direction of its action. Action is directly upon the organism and indirectly upon the poison. Physiological antidoting takes place between drugs according to the law of the Repulsion of Similars.

"Medicines producing similar symptoms are related to each other and are mutually antidotal in proportion to the degree of their symptom-similarity." (Boenninghausen.) Hence, the rule, "Let similars be cured (treated) by similars"—*"Similia Similibus Curentur."*

Chemical antidotes act on the poisons themselves rather than against their effects. Their action depends upon their property of uniting chemically with poisonous substances and altering their chemical and physical character. By their use soluble and absorbable substances are converted into insoluble or partly soluble substances, which may then be removed from the body by physical or other means. Their use is restricted to cases in which the poison is known and capable of being directly acted upon chemically. The remaining dynamical effects of the poison, if any, must still be antidoted dynamically.

So-called "mechanical antidotes," while necessary and useful, do not properly come under the head of antidotes. They are merely means of accomplishing physical expulsion of the poisonous substances from the body, after which dynamical antidotes are required to remove the pathogenetic effects of so much of the poison as has been absorbed, exactly as in cases where chemical antidotes are used.

A true therapeutics, therefore, stands as the connecting link between pathology and pharmacology. Without an adequate therapy, pathology and pharmacology have only an academic interest for students and savants who love to dig curiously into the things of nature. With an adequate and efficient therapeutics they become powerful agencies for benefiting humanity. With a false therapeutics they become a curse to the world through the countless evils of drug addiction, prolonged, perverted and suppressed disease, ruined lives, crippled and mutilated bodies and blasted minds. The shores of time are strewn with pitiful wrecks, victims of false therapeutic systems and methods, "science falsely so-called."

Science is erected upon a foundation of facts, principles and laws. Science is related, systematized knowledge.

A system, to be scientific, must be capable of including, explaining and using all the facts upon which it is based. Its fundamental law or principle must include and be harmonious with all its subordinate and related laws and principles. Its technic or practical methods must be based directly upon and conform to the principles which it seeks to apply. Ethics, it hardly needs to be said, requires that its representative shall consistently "practice what he preaches."

A true science of pathology must include and be able to explain all the symptoms of disease—the finer, subjective individual symptoms as well as the general functional, organic and objective changes that occur in disease.

A true science of therapeutics must correspond and connect at every point with its correlated science of pathology, and be capable of adaptation and application to the needs of individual cases of disease.

The identity of the individual must not be lost in the class. A scientific therapeutic system must be broad enough to cover the needs of the individual as well as the class. It will not do to reject one class of basic phenomena (subjective, for example), and attempt to formulate a system upon the remainder.

Therapeutics, as a science exemplified in homœopathy, rests upon two series of phenomena; the phenomena of diseases and the phenomena of drugs or agents used in the treatment of diseases. These two series of phenomena are connected by a general law. Systematized knowledge of the phenomena of diseases constitutes the science of pathology. Systematized knowledge of the phenomena of drugs constitutes the science of pharmacology. Systematized knowledge of the laws, principles and methods which connect the two sciences constitutes the *science* of therapeutics and the effectual use of these in treating and curing the sick constitutes the *art* of healing, or applied therapeutics.

In a true science of medicine, pathology, therapeutics, pharmacology and toxicology as well as medical, physiological and pharmaceutical chemistry are fundamentally one, in having for their principal object the observation, study and treatment of the effects of all agents which act either pathogenically or therapeutically upon the living organism, whether it be in a mechanical, chemical, electrical or dynamical manner.

One fundamental principle underlies them all—the law of reciprocal action or equivalence.

The law of chemical affinity and definite proportions; the law of physiological or dynamical affinity; the law of assimilation; the law of antidotes or the repulsion of similars (upon which is based the theory of cure) are all phases of the universal law of mutual action, which governs every action that occurs in the universe.

Every agent or stimulus, external to the organism, which has the power to excite a vital reaction in the organism, comes legitimately under the universal law and may be applied for therapeutic purposes in accordance therewith, when the corollaries of the law are known.

Pharmaco-therapeutics finally resolves itself into a process of physiological or dynamical antidoting, based upon the law of attraction, affinity or mutual action and governed by the principle of symptom-similarity.

Predisposing, exciting and contributing causes of disease all come to this in the end—that by some condition or combination of conditions they ultimate in the production of a *poison* the action of which is the proximate, efficient or specific cause of the reaction of the organism which constitute disease.

Hence, diseases always bear the symptomatic likeness of drugs, or poisons. By mechanical dilution and potentiation poisons may be deprived of their lethal qualities and transformed into healing remedies normally assimilable by the sick organism. Similarity of symptoms is, therefore, the natural guide to the curative remedy, as well as to the true diagnosis of the disease, and comparison of symptoms is the process by which the conclusion is reached.

Idiosyncrasy and Drug Diseases.—*In paragraph 30,* Organon, Hahnemann says that medicines *appear* to have a more powerful influence in affecting the health of the body than the natural morbific agencies which produce disease, inasmuch as suitable medicines overcome and cure disease.

In paragraph 31, he remarks that natural disease-producing agencies have only a conditional power of action, depending upon the disposition and degree of susceptibility of the organism. They do not act (perceptibly?) on every one at all times. Of a thousand persons exposed to smallpox, for example, perhaps not more than one or two would be infected, and these only if they happened to be in a susceptible condition at the time of exposure. He implies that the remainder are entirely immune by virtue of natural resistance.

In paragraph 32, he somewhat unguardedly asserts that it is otherwise with drugs; that *they* act unconditionally. Every true medicine, he says, acts at all times, in all persons, under all conditions producing distinctly perceptible symptoms "if the dose be large enough." He here establishes at least one condition. No man in his normal condition is entirely or absolutely immune to a dose of arsenic, or strychnine or quinine, nor to the bacilli of cholera or tuberculosis. *The extent of its action in either case is conditional.* The violence, extent and duration of the effects will be proportionate to the size of the dose and the susceptibility of the individual as influenced by constitution and environment, *but it always acts.* Strictly speaking, every action in the universe is conditional.

One of the problems that frequently confronts the homœopathic physician is how to deal practically with those peculiar and puzzling cases which present the phenomena of what is commonly called idiosyncrasy.

By idiosyncrasy we mean a habit or quality of the organism peculiar to the individual. It is a peculiarity of the constitution, inherited or acquired, which makes the individual morbidly susceptible to some agent or influence which would not so affect others.

To the average physician idiosyncrasy ordinarily means merely an oversensitiveness to some drug. He is called upon, for example, to treat a case of intermittent fever. After giving what he regards as a moderate dose of his favorite quinine he sees his patient quickly become violently delirious; or perhaps develop a violent attack of vomiting and go into collapse; or have a hæmorrhage from the kidneys, or lungs, or into the retina. All these grave conditions have been reported of quinine and some cases with fatal results; or what is nearly as bad, with permanent loss or impairment of function, as blindness, or deafness.

Again he meets a case which seems to require opium. He administers the usual dose and sees it produce dangerous congestion of brain, lungs or intestines. He explains such experiences as being due to idiosyncrasy, substitutes some other drug and lets it go at that. Such experiences do not teach him much and he goes on in the same old way afterward; but there is much to be learned from such cases, if we view them aright.

Other patients manifest a morbid susceptibility to agents and influences not classified as medicinal. For example, a person cannot eat some common article of food without suffering. Apples, peaches, strawberries, fish, shell fish, onions, potatoes, milk, fats or butter, etc., affect certain people unpleasantly in a most peculiar fashion. Then there are the idiosyncrasies of smell. One cannot bear the odor of violets; another of lavender; another of any flowers when he is sick.

One of my patients always gets an attack of hay fever and asthma if he rides behind a horse. The odor and exhalation from a perspiring horse are noxious to him. A woman hay fever victim has a fit of violent trembling and aggravation of all her symptoms if she comes in proximity with a cat. These examples of idiosyncrasy are quite distinct from hysteria and the general oversensitiveness found in neurasthenics and broken-down constitutions, where every little annoyance seems a burden too great to be borne, and every sense is painfully acute.

"The fundamental cause of every idiosyncrasy is morphological unbalance; that is, an organic state in which, through excess and defect in development there results excess and defect in function, with a corresponding degree of hyper-excitability or non-excitability." (Rice.)

Without pausing to set forth more fully the modern scientific explanation of these phenomena we may say that idiosyncrasy, from the standpoint of the homœopathic prescriber, is often the key to a difficult case. Viewed as modalities, these peculiarities, which are merely vagaries to the average practitioner, take on a certain degree of importance as indications for a remedy. Properly interpreted and classified, they sometimes rank as "generals," expressing and representing a peculiarity of the patient himself— of the case as a whole. They aid in individualizing the case and differentiate between two or more similar remedies. Thus, in a certain puzzling case the symptom, "aggravation from onions," discovered only after the case had baffled me for several weeks, led to the selection of Thuja, which cured the case.

Idiosyncrasies are inherited and acquired. They represent a morbid susceptibility to some particular agent or influence. Of their causes there is little more to say, except that the drug idiosyncrasies, both inherited and acquired, appear sometimes to be due to the previous *abuse of the drug,* to which a morbid susceptibility now exists, and that the remainder have their origin in what Hahnemann called the *psoric constitution.* Many persons who have been poisoned by a drug are afterward hypersensitive to that drug—a condition known as anaphylaxis. A familiar example is the susceptibility to Rhus or ivy poisoning of those who have once been poisoned, especially if their initial attack was treated topically, by external remedies. Such persons are poisoned by the slightest contact with the plant, or even by passing in its vicinity without contact. In such cases the disappearance of the original external manifestations of the disease is followed by the setting up of a constitutional susceptibility which renders them peculiarly vulnerable, not only to the particular drug concerned, *but to the diseases to which that drug corresponds homœopathically.* They are illustrations of metastasis, which is regarded by some as being due to a suppression of the primary form of the disease by injudicious topical or palliative treatment. This view is based upon direct observation, and is sustained by analogy with the well-known serious results of the accidental or incidental disappearance or repercussion of external symptoms in the acute eruptive diseases, such as measles and scarlet fever.

Where the initial attack is perfectly cured homœopathically by internal medicines such results never follow. Investigation shows that some cases of inherited idiosyncrasy and morbid susceptibility to drugs are traceable to the abuse of those drugs by parents or ancestors. This relation has been observed particularly in the case of two drugs, sulphur and mercury. A case occurred in my practice in which such a violent and sudden aggravation followed the administration of a high potency of Mercury that the patient's life was endangered. He afterward asked if he had been given mercury, and said that he had never been able to take mercury in any form. He had been salivated by mercury, in youth, and his father and mother before him had been heavy users of the drug. Cases occur in which even amalgam fillings in teeth cause symptoms of mercurial poisoning, from absorption of infinitesimal quantities of mercury.

It has been held that the homœopathic correspondence of sulphur to such a vast number of symptoms and diseases is partly due to the widespread abuse of sulphur by preceding generations; in other words that the commonly found sulphur symptoms which make it curative in so many conditions, represent a vast *proving* of sulphur upon the human race, pursued for several generations, which has created a general morbid susceptibility to the drug. The same might be said of many other drugs, but such an idea, interesting because novel and practically suggestive, should not be given too much weight lest it lead us astray into the realm of speculation.

In the closely related subject of "drug diseases," we are on safer ground. The subject of drug diseases has a particular and perennial interest for the homœopathician, because his professional life is devoted largely to the observation and study of the phenomena produced or cured in the human organism by drugs. It comes before him at every point in his career and he, more clearly than any other, realizes its importance. The homœopathic materia medica, from which he derives his knowledge of the remidies used for the cure of disease, is made up principally of collections of symptoms derived from healthy persons who have intentionally taken small doses of drugs and carefully observed and recorded their effects under the direction of trained observers.

Every proving is the clinical record of an artificial disease produced by some drug. Every case of sickness demands its corresponding drug, which is found by comparing the symptoms of a patient and the symptoms of drugs. For every disease arising from natural causes there has been found, or may be produced by some drug, a similar artificial disease, symptom corresponding with symptom, often to the minutest details. This similar corresponding drug, once found and administered in the proper dose, proves to be the curative. Upon this easily demonstrable fact is founded the homœopathic healing art. From this fact was deduced the healing principle, which is the scientific basis of homœopathy.

Acceptance of the idea that disease may be cured by drugs is quite general, but the truth of the related idea that drugs also *cause disease,* and each drug its own specific disease, although partially recognized, is by no means as clearly recognized as it should be. The alcoholic, the drug addict and the "dope fiend," have long been regarded as "victims of *a disease,*" by some regarded as a peculiar psychical disease and by others in other ways; but only very recently has it dawned upon a few of the "regular" profession that the mysterious, indefinite disease from which the addicts suffer is, in each case, a definite, specific *drug* disease, caused by and representing the action of the particular drug to which he is addicted; that the opium addict suffers from the *opium disease,* the "coke fiend" from the *cocaine disease,* etc.

Homœopathy should have taught them this long ago. Few seem to realize that a very large part of the disease met with in ordinary practice is the result of what may be called involuntary poisoning. Symptoms are constantly appearing in our clinical records which are the product of drugs, either self-administered or ignorantly prescribed by that class of physicians who are forever prescribing for the results of their own drugging without knowing it. There are many, even in the homœopathic school, who do not realize this fact and who fail to see that the problem before them is as often one of antidoting a drug as of curing a true natural disease. This has a very practical bearing on the case, for the first step in such cases is to seek out and stop the use of drugs and antidote them, rather than to blindly proceed to give more drugs. Nature unaided will often remove many of the symptoms in such cases if the dosing is stopped and a little time is given. The remainder becomes the basis of homœopathic prescribing under accepted homœopathic principles, and the case as a whole affords an opportunity for the discerning physician to impart some wholesome instruction in the rules of right living.

Hering said: "The last taken drug affords the best indication for the next prescription." The experienced homœopathic physician, therefore, gives particular attention in the examination of cases to ascertaining what drugs have been previously used, with a view to stopping their use and antidoting such as have been most influential in producing disorder, as revealed by a study of the symptoms.

Over-dosing and too frequent changing of remedies in homœopathic practice often leads to the confusion of the prescriber and the damage of the patient.

This was exemplified in a case seen by me in consultation with a young physician. The patient was an infant about eighteen months old who had been under treatment for two weeks. The diagnosis was indefinite, because the nature of the initial disease was obscure. The case did not at first seem serious and probably was not; but the child was now obviously very sick and there had been no signs of improvement. The young physician exhibited his up-to-date card record of the case, very neatly kept. It contained the symptoms of the first examination, quite fully and clearly taken, with temperatures, pulse and respiration carefully charted. The first prescription was Belladonna 3x, which manifestly as to remedy, if not to dose, corresponded closely to the symptoms as recorded and was a good prescription. But the record showed that on his visit the following day, finding his patient slightly worse, he had changed the prescription and given two other rem-

GENERAL PATHOLOGY OF HOMŒOPATHY

edies, also in very low dilutions, in alternation. From that time on the prescription was changed almost daily, two remedies in alternation being given each time and presently, palliatives and adjuvants, cathartics, stimulants, etc., began to show on the record. In the two weeks of treatment some twenty different medicines had been given, in strength ranging from mother tincture to 3x dilution. The result, of course, was inevitable. Given the sensitive organism of an infant, acted upon by such a number of medicines but slightly removed by dilution from the crude state, each one being capable of exciting more or less toxic reaction, and one could surely foretell the result—"confusion worse confounded." *Every drug given had produced some effect,* if not the effect desired. The resulting symptom picture was of the well-known "composite" character, blurred and indefinite, with little or no character. Hardly one clear-cut, definite symptom could be found—much less that group of consistent and co-ordinated symptoms which is required in making an accurate homœopathic prescription. It was a clear case of getting lost in a very small patch of woods. If the doctor, after making his first prescription to Bell. 3x had known how to rightly interpret the fact that the patient seemed *somewhat worse the next day* instead of better, as he had expected; if he had then discontinued the remedy without giving anything else except placebo and awaited the curative reaction, he would have found his patient much improved on the following day. Without knowing it he was then witnessing that "slight aggravation of the symptoms" following the exhibition of a well-selected remedy of which Hahnemann warns us. Better still would it have been if he had given the Belladonna in the thirtieth or two hundredth potency in the first instance, instead of the 3x. There would then have been no aggravation, the patient would have been better on the second day, and would probably have gone on to rapid recovery. Instead of this, however, the doctor misinterpreted the facts, thereby doing himself, his patient and homœopathy injustice. Believing that he had made a wrong prescription, he changed it. In his beginning confusion he further departed from sound principles by giving two medicines in alternation, thus multiplying the sources of error and confusion. From this point on, like a man lost in the woods, he was simply "walking circles around himself"—hopelessly lost as far as his own efforts were concerned, until somebody came and guided him home.

The toxic effects of drugs prescribed in the ordinary routine of practice are commonly overlooked. In spite of a popular delusion to the contrary, a drug loses none of its power in being prescribed by a man who writes M. D. after his name. Today, as in the dark ages, there are physicians who give drugs as if they believed that each of them at their behest, would find its way through the devious channels of the body and perform the exact task assigned to it. Unlike the chemist and the pork packer, they do not see the "by-products," nor make use of them.

It was said of the pork packers that they had learned to utilize every part of the pig except his squeal. Then came an enterprising phonograph firm whose agents invaded the slaughter house and actually recorded the squeals for reproduction, thus completing the work of salvage.

It is different with the doctors. If the patient recovers after his dosing all is well and the doctor is confirmed in his faith. If the patient gets worse, or new symptoms arise, all is still well, medically speaking. It is merely a "complication" for which he has a ready name and a convenient pathological classification. If the patient dies there is no lack of causes assignable on a pathological basis, and the requirements of the Health Department are easily met in filling the blanks in the death certificate. Thus "science" is vindicated and the doctor felicitates himself on his diagnostic and pathological acumen. His faith in drugs is not shaken.

Rarely does it occur to the prescriber that the "complication" is but the symptomatic reflection of the drug or drugs he has previously given. Sometimes he does seem to have faint glimpses of that unpleasant truth, as when tetanus, trismus or acute Bright's disease speedily follow vaccination; or when hæmorrhage in lungs, kidneys or retina quickly supervenes upon the administration of massive doses of quinine; or when he happens to recognize one of the "puzzling eruptions" said to be caused by one or more of the twenty-nine drugs named by Glentworth Butler, in his work, "The Diagnostics of Internal Medicine." But such flashes of insight are rare and accomplish little in stemming the tide of drugs which is engulfing so many victims. Though such a physician may be as keen on the scent of the last new bacillus as Buster was on the trail of Bunny Cottontail, his nose is singularly dull when it comes to trailing the *most common of all causes of disease*—the preceding drug.

In the rank and file of medicine the old ideas on pharmacology still obtain, in spite of vaunted progress. A drug, or combination of drugs, when administered to a patient, is supposed to have no other effects than those assigned theoretically to the class to which it belongs. The "other effects," which are sure to arise, are attributed to the natural progress of the disease or to some theoretical "complication."

When we come to examine these allopathic drug classifications from the standpoint of that knowledge of drugs which is derived from actual observation of their effects upon the healthy, as recorded in homœopathic provings, we find them to be of the crudest character, based upon the most superficial knowledge of drug action. The gross toxic effects of the drug, as observed accidentally in men or animals or as guessed, are set over against equally crude generalizations of diseases, usually on the antipathic principle where any principle at all is discoverable.

For although the allopathic school of medicine of the present day repudiates any law or principle, it is plain that the rule of contraries still dominates it. One has only to take down any standard allopathic work on materia medica to find its drugs arranged in some twenty-five or thirty classes, the names of which either begin with "anti" or imply the same thing, as pointed out by the late Dr. Conrad Wesselhoeft, of Boston. Thus we find anti-toxins, anti-spasmodics, anti-periodics, anti-pyretics, anti-acids, anti-septics, anthelmintics, alteratives, tonics, counter-irritants, etc. Manifestly, the appellation "allopathy" holds good today, as it did a hundred years ago, when Hahnemann applied it.

As long as drugs retain their power to make well people sick, and as long as doctors continue to make such generalizations as these, so long must both be recognized and dealt with as causative factors in the production of human ills. And so, as our allopathic neighbors and our homœopathic brethren with allopathic proclivities remain as yet in a large majority, there will continue to be plenty of work for the real followers of Hahnemann to do in dealing with the results of their medical obtuseness for some time to come. True it is that if the use of crude drugs could be entirely done away with, the sum of human ills would be greatly reduced; or, as Dr. Oliver Wendell Holmes wittily said: "If all the drugs in the world were dumped into the sea, it would be better for mankind *and the worse for the fishes."* In either case probably two-thirds of the existing ornaments of the medical profession would shine in other spheres with at least equal radiance.

This phase of the subject is important from a practical standpoint. Cases will frequently present themselves which are puzzling, and resist all efforts to cure until they are recognized as "drug cases." The trouble may be entirely due to drugs, or there may be a combination in varying proportions of drug and disease symptoms.

It should be a matter of routine in making first examinations, to ascertain what drugs have been used. In chronic cases this investigation should extend back through the whole life-time of the patient. The diseases from which the patient has suffered, and the drugs used in their treatment should be ascertained if possible. The patient may not know all, but he will usually know some of the most common and powerful drugs he has taken, and a search of the druggists' files may reveal the rest. The key to a difficult case may be the drug or drugs which have "cured" some acute disease, perhaps early in the patient's medical history. Antidoting the drug clears up the case.

Frequently, for example, will some chronic disease of the liver, kidneys, spleen or lungs be traced back to an initial attack of malarial fever checked by massive doses of quinine or arsenic. The patient has "never been well since." The seemingly indicated remedies do not act. A few doses of the appropriate antidote, perhaps Arnica, or Ipecac, or Pulsatilla, or even of Arsenic or Cinchona—the abused drugs themselves, *in high potency*—will clear up the case and either cure or render it amenable to other symptomatically indicated drugs.

It is a fact that the high potency of a drug is sometimes the best antidote for the effects of the crude drug.

It is not unusual in the treatment of such cases for the original symptoms to be reproduced. I have seen a full-fledged, typical attack of intermittent fever reproduced in a case which had become tubercular, within a week after the administration of an antidotal dose of Arsenic in high potency. The patient made a rapid recovery. The initial attack of intermittent fever, in the case referred to, was five years before.

In a case variously diagnosed as "chronic gout," "chronic articular rheumatism," etc., unsuccessfully treated by many physicians, including European specialists, I witnessed the reappearance of a discharge from the urethra fifteen years after the original gonorrhœal discharge had disappeared under the influence of astringent injections. With the establishment of the discharge the patient's "rheumatic" symptoms began to rapidly improve and a perfect cure resulted. This was a case of chronic gonococcic septicæmia, or so-called "gonorrhœal rheumatism," in reality, metastasis of the original disease caused by the use of injections. The key which unlocked the door and released the imprisoned disease was Thuja, the typical "anti-sycotic" remedy of Hahnemann.

Drug symptoms and complications often arise in the most unexpected and surprising ways, and baffle all but the most acute and experienced examiners. Hair dyes and tonics, complexion beautifiers, dentifrices, medicated soaps, antiseptics; borax in baby's mouth to prevent sprue, and carbolic acid in mama's douche to prevent babies; innumerable ointments and lotions; to say nothing about the equally numerous patent and proprietary nostrums which fill the shelves of the corner drug stores and find their way "down the red lane" into the human system, all play their part in creating morbid susceptibility, idiosyncrasy and drug diseases and in making work for the doctor.

These are some of the things to look for among the possible causes of a disease. They are things very generally overlooked by that type of physician who either does not know their importance, will not take the time and pains to find out, or does not care. The patients of such physicians are fair game for the man who does know, who will take the time, and who does care; and he will not be in practice very long before he bags his share of them.

CHAPTER IX

Cure and Recovery

The Recall of the Medical Profession.—The advent of homœopathy in the world opened a new era in medicine and gave new meaning to the word "Cure." In the Organon of Medicine, Hahnemann, in military parlance, "sounded the recall" to all physicians in the field and laid before them a new plan of campaign and a new method of attack upon the enemy forces of disease. For the first time in history it then became possible to treat diseases under scientific principles and perform true cures by medication.

The New Ideal.—Hahnemann contemplated the entire field of medicine from the standpoint of an ideal and efficient therapeutics. In the first paragraph of the Organon he penetrated directly to the heart of the matter and declared that the "physician's high and only mission is to restore the sick to health—to cure."

Here Hahnemann took his stand. From this point he viewed his field. By this standard he measured all physicians, all medical theories, methods and systems and he desired and demanded the same measurement for himself and his own method. He asked but one question, applied but one test, *Do they cure the sick?* Experience and observation of the men and methods of his day showed clearly that they did not cure. In the light of a vast and comprehensive knowledge and a bitterly disappointing personal experience, he pronounced the medicine of his day a failure and set about its reformation.

Cure was not then, as it has since become in the dominant school of medicine, an obsolete term. Physicians still talked and wrote of "cures," but vainly sought to find them. "The Art of Healing" or "The Healing Art" were familiar phrases, but the thing itself, like a will-o'-the-wisp, eluded them—then as it has ever since.

In the second paragraph of the Organon, Hahnemann gives, for the first time in medical history, an adequate and satisfying definition of the ideal expressed in the word "Cure:" "The highest ideal of a cure is rapid, gentle and permanent restoration of health, or removal and annihilation of the disease in its whole extent, in the shortest, most reliable and most harmless way, *on easily comprehensible principles.*"

Principles, not Precedents.—In those last four words lies the main point of the whole matter. Cure is dependent, not upon precedent, opinion or speculation but upon the application of *Principles;* principles, moreover, that are "easily comprehensible." The only principles that are easily comprehensible are principles that *are true*. The only principles that are true are principles logically deduced from facts—*all the facts* that belong to the field of research involved. Simplicity—comprehensibility—is the highest criterion of Truth. The greatest truths are always simple.

Medicine in general and therapeutics in particular are authoritatively classified among the Arts.

From time immemorial the practice of medicine has been called "The Art of Healing," hence, a cure is a product of art. Let us consider what is meant by Art.

Art Defined.—Art is practice *guided by correct principles* in the use of means for the attainment of a desired end.

An artist is one who is skilled in applying knowledge or ability to the accomplishment of a concrete purpose.

Psychologically, art is the superior work of reason and intelligence, actuated by a sense of beauty and the "eternal fitness of things."

Art transcends nature. It represents the victory of mind over matter, of man over nature. The Artist can take a hint from nature and devise some quicker or better way of accomplishing certain purposes; as when the homœopathic artist takes the crude materials that nature provides and adapts them directly to therapeutic ends by potentiation, rendering them harmless, more active, more potent, more assimilable and hence more efficient.

Art not Imitation of Nature.—Art is not mere servile imitation of nature, nor of nature's processes, although such base imitations are constantly being foisted upon the medical profession and the public in the name of art or science.

Hahnemann says: "The vital force, capable only of acting in

harmony with the physical arrangement of our organism, and without reason, insight or reflection, was not given to us that we should regard it as the best guide in the cure of disease. What man of sense would undertake to *imitate nature* in her endeavors of coming to the rescue. . . . No, the true healing art is that *intellectual office* incumbent on *the higher human mind* and *free powers of thought,* discriminating and deciding *according to cause.*"

To illustrate: Many examples of the working of the homœopathic principle may be found in nature: The happy but unexpected results of accidental experiences, such as relief from rubbing a bruise, applying snow to a frozen ear, or radiant heat to a burned finger; the instinctive actions of sick or injured animals, as when they eat grass or leaves to produce vomiting when they are nauseated, or lick the secretions from their own wounds or sores.

If a homœopathic artist desired to profit by the observation that a dog had apparently cured himself by licking the pus from his own sores, or that a human victim of septicæmia had recovered after accidentally or intentionally ingesting a portion of his own morbid secretions, he would not think of imitating these procedures. Desiring to ascertain the value of "autogenous pus" as a possible remedy, he would first submit the morbid product to the recognized scientific process of modification by mechanical potentiation, according to the method of Hahnemann and carry it to a point where there could be no question of the non-existence of toxic or septic qualities.

Having thus removed the obnoxious qualities of the substance and raised it from the physical to the dynamical plane, he would next submit it to the test of proving upon healthy persons; or, if he chose to approach the problem first from the clinical side he would administer doses of the potentiated substance to the person from whom it was taken and observe results, checking them up later by the results of a proving.

To illustrate: Venomous reptiles and insects inject their poison by puncturing the skin and obtain quick and positive results. This suggests but does not justify the use of the hypodermic needle for therapeutic purposes, than which no more pernicious violation of the principles of true medical art was ever devised.

The use of the hypodermic needle for therapeutic purposes is merely a slavish imitation of nature, and of nature in her most malignant moods. The avowed object of the procedure is to get "quick" and "positive" results, but like many other questionable medical expedients, it is a violation of the principles of the healing art and an evil to be combated by every homœopathician.

If every hypodermic needle in existence were destroyed it would still be possible to cure or relieve every curable disease quickly and safely, by means of the appropriate medicine administered by the natural channels.

Imitation of nature is a paltry substitute for art. Whatever may be the outcome in the long run and final accounting, nature, temporarily at least, works irrationally, blindly, painfully and wastefully; as when she creates a million spawn to secure a dozen fish; or suppurates an eye away in the effort to remove a splinter from the cornea. Undoubtedly law underlies all such efforts, but it is a law violated, thwarted or hampered in its operations by adverse conditions. Art thereupon steps in, removes obstacles, quiets disturbance, improves conditions and accomplishes results *with the least expenditure of force,* by means perhaps similar, but always superior to those used by nature.

Cure is never accomplished by methods which are but a mere imitation of nature or nature's processes. Recoveries, only, result from such methods. Frequently great injury is inflicted upon the patient by the use of such methods, because many of nature's processes cannot be successfully imitated by man. There is always something which eludes us in our attempt to grasp nature's deeper secrets.

Distinction Between Cure and Recovery. The favorable outcome of medical treatment may be either a *cure* or a *recovery.* To realize the ideal of cure, it is necessary to know the exact meaning of these terms and to be able to discriminate between them.

Failure to discriminate between cure and recovery engenders confusion of thought and leads to pernicious practices. The terms are not synonymous. Natural recoveries following treatment consisting of mere palliation of symptoms should not be mistaken for cures nor falsely paraded as such. In either case, a false standard is set up, injustice is done to the ideal of cure and scientific progress is retarded.

A Cure is Always a Result of Art and is Never Brought About by Nature.—Nature, however, aided or unaided, often brings about a recovery, under the operation of natural laws. Fortunate indeed is it for humanity that this is true.

Aside from homœopathy, sanitation and surgery, the only real progress in handling the problem of disease during the last century has been in the adoption of hygienic methods of treatment tending toward natural recovery—the abolition of all drugs and dependence upon rest, diet, regimen and good nursing—known as the expectant method. The rate of mortality in certain diseases has fallen in proportion to the degree that meddlesome medication has been superseded by sound hygienic methods.

Definition of Recovery.—Recovery is the spontaneous return of the patient to health after the removal, disappearance or cessation of the exciting causes and occasion of disease, or as a result of treatment which is not directly and specifically curative in its nature.

Recovery takes place by virtue of the existence of sufficient integrity of organs and inherent power of reaction in the patient to overcome the disease-producing agency without the aid of the homœopathic or healing art. Recovery is favored by the application of sound principles of mental and physical hygiene, judicious mechanical or surgical treatment when required, avoidance of drugs used for their "physiological" (really pathogenic) effects, and by enlightened sanitation.

The Expectant Treatment Inadequate.—Nature unaided, however, or with all the aid afforded by the expectant treatment and by sanitation and surgery, is unable to cope successfully with many forms of severe disease. Such diseases as cholera, yellow fever, pneumonia, diphtheria, typhus and typhoid fever, smallpox, and many other diseases take a heavy toll in mortality, practically uninfluenced by the expectant treatment, except as compared with the much greater mortality under ordinary drug treatment. If diseases are divided into three classes with regard to their rate of mortality, the highest mortality is found among those treated by ordinary drug methods, the next lower under the expectant method, and the lowest under homœopathic treatment.

The Superiority of Homœopathy.—Homœopathy has gained

its greatest triumphs in those diseases which are uninfluenced by even the expectant treatment. Of these cholera is a notable example. With a normal mortality of from forty to seventy per cent. under any other form of treatment, the mortality under homœopathic treatment, but otherwise under precisely the same general conditions, has been as low as four per cent. Substantially the same is true of other diseases, in all of which the mortality is distinctly lower under homœopathic treatment than under the expectant treatment, which is itself so superior to ordinary drug treatment that the leaders of thought and research in the regular school warmly advocate the abandonment of all drugs except mercury, quinin and morphin in special cases.

It is the duty of every physician to avail himself of all the resources of hygiene, sanitation and surgery, but it is also his duty to put prejudice aside and investigate the claims of a method of medication which can show such markedly superior results as does homœopathy.

Homœopathy alone, of all therapeutic methods, can legitimately claim to effect true cures by medication, as distinguished from recoveries; and this it claims, first, because it is based upon a definite general principle or law of nature; second, because it is able to successfully apply that principle to individual cases; and third, because it does actually restore the sick to health, quickly, safely, gently and permanently, upon easily comprehensible principles.

Relation of Cure to Disease.—A true definition of cure must be based upon a right conception of the nature of disease.

The Standard Dictionary defines disease as "any departure from, failure in, or perversion of normal physiological *action* in the material constitution or *functional* integrity of the living organism."

This definition rightly focuses attention upon the dynamical aspect of the subject, for disease is essentially and primarily a morbid dynamical disturbance of the vital powers and functions, resulting in a loss of functional and organic balance.

Primarily and essentially, cure is the restoration directly, by medical art, or normal physiological action. Cures do not consist in the mere removal of the external, secondary, tangible products of disease, but in restoration of the dynamical balance, so that the functions of the organism are again performed normally and the patient is in a state of health.

Disease is manifested perceptibly by signs and symptoms. Cure is manifested by the removal of the symptoms. Strictly speaking the removal of all the symptoms of the case is equivalent to a cure, but if symptoms disappear and the patient is not restored to health and strength it means either that some of the most important symptoms of the case have been overlooked, or that the case has passed beyond the curable stage. All curable cases present perceptible symptoms, but their discernment often depends upon the acuteness of the observer.

Cure relates to the case as a whole: A patient may have his hæmorrhoids removed and be relieved of his rectal symptoms; but if the symptoms of the heart or liver disease which preceded and caused his hæmorrhoids are not removed the patient is not cured; and so of innumerable other morbid conditions. Cure refers to *the patient,* not to some symptoms of his disease, nor to what may be called "one of his diseases." To say that a patient is cured of his hæmorrhoids, but still has his heart disease is absurd. Cure means complete restoration to health.

Cure is not affected by the removal surgically nor by any local means, of the external, secondary, pathological "end-products" of disease, such as tumors, effusions, collections of pus, useless organs or dead tissues; *for the morbid functioning which produced those effects often remains unchanged, after such removal.*

Cure is effected only by dynamical treatment according to fixed principles, directed to the primary, functional disorder as revealed by the complete symptom-picture preceding and accompanying the formation of the tangible products of the disease.

Cure is not merely the removal of the *primary causes of disease,* for even if all the causes of the disease are known and removable, the effects, having been begun, may continue as secondary causes after the removal of the primary causes. Spontaneous disappearance of the disease does not always occur in such cases, and dynamical treatment is required to restore the patient to health.

The End Products of Disease and Mechanical Treatment.

—The tangible, physical results of disease as thus defined may and often do disappear spontaneously when the internal dynamic disturbance is removed by curative medication, but they are not primarily the object of homœopathic treatment. It may be necessary eventually, to remove them mechanically by surgical art. Surgical or mechanical measures become necessary when the tangible products of disease are so far advanced or so highly developed that they become secondary causes of disease and obstacles to cure. In all cases in which disease has ultimated in organic or tissue changes which have progressed to a point where surgical interference is necessary, homœopathic dynamical treatment should precede and follow operation; bearing in mind always that such changes are the direct result of preceding and accompanying morbid functional changes, and that the patient is not cured unless normal functioning is restored.

The Object of Treatment.—The primary object or purpose of homœopathic treatment is the restoration of normal functional balance—health.

The basis of the homœopathic prescription is the totality of the symptoms which represent the functional disorder—*the abnormal process of the disease itself,* not its ultimates or "end-products."

The physician who prescribes for a tumor or any other tangible product of disease is misdirecting his energies and courting failure.

Physicians are constantly mistaking the *product* for the *process* of disease. The product can only be changed by changing the process. Destroying the product does not change the process. Correct the faulty process and the product will take care of itself, so far as homœopathy is concerned. This defines the sphere of homœopathy and this is what we mean when we say that the cure of disease is a dynamical problem.

A Law of Cure Implied.—The accomplishment of even one true cure by medication implies the existence of a governing principle or law of cure by medication. The occasional occurrence of accidental cures very early attracted the attention of medical men and led them to seek for such a law. Glimpses of the law were had by individuals from time to time down the ages, but it eluded the searches or failed of demonstration until Hahnemann finally grasped it comprehendingly and made it the basis for the therapeutic method which he named homœopathy.

Many were deluded by mistaking natural recoveries for cures. Their attempts to "imitate" invariably failed. Others abandoned the idea of a general principle of cure by medication and denied its existence, refusing to accept the demonstration when it was finally made. That is the attitude of the average member of the dominant school to-day. He denies the existence of a general principle of therapeutic medication. "We do not profess a cure," he says; "we only aid nature to bring about recoveries." In this he is at least honest, and consistent in his use of terms.

The Requirements of Cure.—The first requirement of a cure by medication is that it shall be *the result of the direct application of a definite general principle of therapeutic medication.* The result may be accidental or intentional on the part of the prescriber in a given case, but its relation to the means employed must be capable of rational explanation and demonstration by reference to the governing principle.

A general principle is capable of systematic demonstration, not only once but repeatedly and invariably, under stated conditions. Given the principle, it is always possible to formulate a method or technic, by means of which the principle may be successfully applied to every case within its scope.

The second requirement of a cure by medication is that it must be individual. A general principle according to which any action takes place is always capable of being individualized. The ability to meet the varying requirements of individual cases proves the existence and truth of the principle involved.

A true system of therapeutics must be able to adapt its basic principle and its remedy to the needs of each individual case.

There are no cures for "diseases," no remedy for all cases of the same disease. Cure relates to the individual patient, not to the disease. No two cases of the same disease are exactly alike. Differences of manifestation in symptoms and modalities always exist in individuals. It is these differences which give each case its individuality, and create the need for an individual remedy.

The Morphological Factor.—Every individual develops

according to a certain morphological tendency or predisposition, inherent in his constitution. It is from this tendency that he derives his individuality. This tendency or predisposition may be or become morbid. If it does, the symptomatic form of that morbidity will also be individual. It is necessary, therefore, to study each case of disease from the morphological as well as the semeiological standpoint in order to be able to determine its individual form and characteristics.

The new morphology includes all the facts and phenomena, anatomical, physiological and psychological, functional and organic, normal or abnormal, which represent the individuality of the subject. It aims to establish in each concrete case the particular kind or variety of organization, development and functioning which gives it individuality and differentiates it from other similar cases, thus providing a reliable basis for the rational interpretation of symptoms and the selection of the remedy indicated for the patient.

The Examination of the Patient and Construction of the Case.—Disease is primarily a dynamical disturbance of the vital functions of the individual organism, manifesting itself by signs and symptoms. Symptoms are the only perceptible evidence of disease and the only guide to the curative medicine. For the prescriber the characteristic symptoms of each individual in the totality constitute the disease and their removal is the object of treatment and the cure.

The third requirement for the performance of an ideal cure, therefore, is a complete and impartial collection and record of the facts which constitute the natural and medical history of the individual.

This should include not only physical and constitutional signs, the heredity and family history of the patient; how he was born, raised and educated; his occupation, habits, social and domestic relations; but a chronological symptomatic history of all his diseases, indispositions, idiosyncrasies, accidents and vicissitudes, as far as they can be recalled.

In considering the recorded results of each examination, the homœopathic therapeutist pays particular attention to the unusual, peculiar, exceptional features or symptoms which give the case its individuality; for, by these, under the guidance of the principle of symptom-similarity, he is led to the remedy needed for the cure of the individual case.

Symptoms, general and particular, "behave themselves in a particular way," take on peculiar forms, combinations and modalities, according to the morphological type, environment, personality and predisposition of the individual.

It is necessary thus to study the individual in order to understand how a general or particular predisposition to disease becomes concrete and the object of treatment and cure, as well as to elicit the symptoms which are to guide in the selection of the remedy.

Manner and Direction of Cure.—Cures take place in a definite, orderly manner and direction.

Normal vital processes, cellular, organic and systemic, begin at the center and proceed outwardly. Figuratively, if not literally, life is a centrifugal force, radiating, externalizing, concentrating and organizing spirit into matter—"from above, downward." In the same sense disease is a centripetal force, opposing, obstructing, penetrating toward the center and tending to disorganization.

The progression of all chronic diseases is from the surface toward the center; from less important to more important organs—"from below upward."

Curative medicines reinforce the life force, reverse the morbid process and annihilate the disease. Symptoms disappear from above downward, from within outward and in the reverse order of their appearance.

When a patient with an obscure rheumatic endocarditis, for example, begins to have signs and symptoms of acute arthritis soon after taking the homœopathic remedy and is relieved of his chest sufferings, we know that cure has commenced.

Cure takes place in much less time than natural recovery, without pain, physiological disturbance or danger from the use of the remedy employed and without sequelæ. The restoration of health is complete and lasting.

The Trend of Modern Therapeutics.—Cure, as a medical ideal, appears to have been abandoned by the dominant school of medicine. Formerly, every new therapeutic method or measure based its claims to acceptance upon alleged cures. If the results of its use could be made to pass for cures, it was given some sort of standing in the medical world. If not, or if time revealed the falsity of the claim, it was relegated to the limbo of exploded theories.

With the progress of science and the general diffusion of knowledge, both profession and people have begun to realize their mistakes. A great majority of the alleged cures are found to be not cures at all, but, at best, only recoveries. In many cases, the condition of the patient after his supposed cure is found to be worse than it was before, for the removal or suppression of some of his superficial symptoms, which was all that was accomplished, was followed by other symptoms indicating the invasion of deeper and more important organs by metastasis. The young man, for instance, whose gonorrhœa was treated by injections, and who was told by his physician, after the discharge disappeared, that he was cured and might marry the girl of his choice, soon found that his previously healthy young wife began to complain of serious trouble in her reproductive organs. He found himself watching the gradual fading of the roses in her cheeks and the brightness in her eyes; her lassitude, failing strength and falling weight; her mental depression and irritability; until, finally, consultation with a gynæcologist and a physical examination revealed a gonococcic salpingitis, "a pus tube" or a degenerated ovary, for which the only recourse is an operation and removal of the diseased organs. Result, a mutilated and crippled reproductive organism and a farewell to all hopes of a family. The young man learned too late that he was never cured of his gonorrhœa, but that the measures used merely drove the disease to deeper parts, from whence it was communicated to his innocent wife with such dire results.

Seventy-five per cent. of the alarmingly large and increasing number of operations on the female sexual organs are said by high authorities to be due to chronic gonococcic infection, caused by suppression (by local treatment) and metastasis of the acute disease in the husband. It is a sad commentary on the boasted efficiency of modern therapeutics.

Examples in many forms of disease might be given to illustrate the results of a false and pernicious therapeutics and ignorance of what cure really means; but enough has been said to indicate the importance of a reëxamination of the subject.

The abandonment of the ideal of cure by the general profession and the disappearance of the term from current medical literature does not mean that cure is impossible. It only means that the wrong method has been pursued in the effort to attain it.

Many great truths have had their rise, acceptance and period of sway, followed by a long period of decline and obscurity; but never has a great truth been lost. There is always a "Remnant in Israel" who survive to hold the truth committed to them as a precious possession and cherish it until a revival comes.

The Hahnemannian ideal of cure by medication, according to the principle of symptom-similarity, largely lost sight of for a time in the dazzling accomplishments of modern surgery and laboratory research, has been passing through such a period of neglect and obscurity. But already there are signs of a revival of this great truth, as science, in its wider reaches, is beginning to correlate the results of its work. The whole trend of modern medical thought is toward the confirmation and acceptance of fundamental postulates and principles first enunciated by Hahnemann. Homœopathy is gradually being rediscovered by modern science.

CHAPTER X

INDISPOSITIONS AND THE SECOND BEST REMEDY

Not every case which presents itself to the physician requires medicine. It may only require the searching out and correcting of some evil habit, some error in the mode of living, such as faulty diet, unsanitary surroundings, non-observance of ordinary hygienic requirements in regard to breathing, exercise, sleeping, etc.

In Par. 4 of the *Organon,* Hahnemann says: "He (the physician) is likewise a preserver of health if he knows the things that derange health and cause disease, and how to remove them from persons in health."

In Par. 5 the physician is enjoined to search out "the most probable exciting cause of the acute disease, as also the most significant points in the whole history of the chronic disease to enable him to discover its *fundamental cause,* which is generally due to a chronic miasm."

In making these investigations he directs our attention to "the *physical constitution* of the patient, his moral and intellectual character, his occupation, mode of living and habits, his social and domestic relations, his age, sexual functions, etc."

But this line of investigation is equally fruitful and necessary in dealing with the indispositions of which I am particularly speaking.

In the note to Par. 7, Hahnemann says: "As a matter of course every sensible physician will remove such causes at first, after which the indisposition will generally cease spontaneously." By way of illustration he goes on to say: "He will remove from the room strong smelling flowers, which have a tendency to cause syncope and hysterical sufferings;" (and I may add that he will order hysterical and neurotic "lady patients" to abandon the use of the strong perfumes and sachet bags with which they render the air of their rooms unfit to breathe, aggravate their complaints and make themselves a nuisance to everyone who comes near them); "extract from the cornea the foreign body that excites inflammation of the eye; loosen the over-tight bandage on a wounded limb, ligature the wounded artery, promote the expulsion of poisonous ingesta by vomiting, extract foreign substances from the orifices of the body, crush or remove vesical calculi, open the imperforate anus of the new born infant, etc."

In short, Hahnemann has done his best to make it clear that the use of *common sense* is not incompatible with homœopathic practice, his enemies and some of his overzealous followers to the contrary notwithstanding.

The young homœopathic doctor, fresh from the halls of materia medica, with his brand new case of medicines, is apt to be like the small boy with his first jack-knife who wants to carve and whittle everything within reach—a simile, by the way, quite as applicable to the young surgeon! Both of them leave a trail which to follow does not require the sagacity of a Sherlock Holmes.

Consider for a few moments, then, that class of cases which require for their use only the correction of faulty habits and the removal of exciting causes. Consider also that it often requires the exhibition of as much wisdom, skill, good judgment and *tact* to perform this function as it does to prescribe medicine; indeed, it often requires more. It is much easier to deal out medicine and dismiss the patient, than it is to make a careful investigation of the habits and circumstances of a patient who probably does not need medicine at all, but only wise and kindly advice on how to live.

Great is the power and value of homœopathic medicine, but, like all other good things, it can be abused. Even high potencies can be abused and cause mischief, as I saw illustrated very strikingly when I was sent for in haste to see a patient for whom I had prescribed a few days before. I relate the case because it not only illustrates the particular point I am discussing now, but also the subject of posology which I shall take up subsequently. The patient was an old gentleman who was in a state of mild senile dementia, with enfeebled power of thought, loss of memory, tendency to involuntary urination and defæcation, rather persistent sleeplessness, and becoming careless in his personal habits. But he had been perfectly tractable and mild in his demeanor, and had made no trouble for his family. The symptoms led me to prescribe a remedy, which I gave in the two hundredth potency, with directions to take two doses daily. Three days later I was sent for in haste to see him. I found him in a highly excited state of mind, with flushed face, widely dilated pupils, staring expression and suspicious of being poisoned. He excitedly and harshly accused me of giving him "another man's medicine" which had "filled his bowels up;" he had removed all his clothes, refused to put them on again, and was going about the house nude before the women, without shame, and had tried to go out of doors in that state.

I recognized the symptoms immediately, as I hope you have done. Probably most of you will be able to name the remedy. It was Hyosciamus, of course.

On making inquiries I found that instead of taking the remedy twice a day as directed, owing to a misunderstanding, he had been taking it *every two hours*. Of course he was making a proving—of *the two hundredth potency!* A single dose of Belladonna, two hundredth, removed the whole trouble in a few hours, and he resumed his ordinary placid course of life.

An experience of that kind has a strong tendency to remove any scepticism one may have as to the power of high potencies. It also conveys an impressive warning against too frequent repetition of doses. Moreover, it upsets the theory that high potencies do not act upon the aged. Incidentally it shows the possibility, sometimes denied, of making provings with highly potentiated medicines and substantiates the claims of those who hold that no remedy can be considered as well proved until it has been proved in the potencies as well as in crude form.

It is well known that the most valuable part of a drug action, the finer shadings of symptomatology, are almost never brought out under the use of the tinctures and low potencies. These appear usually under the action of a medium or high potency, or toward the close of a proving of a low potency, long after the first effects of the drug have passed away; so that it has come to be a maxim among experienced provers that *the last appearing symptoms in a proving are the most valuable and characteristic.* In the same way, the *last appearing symptoms in a disease,* especially chronic disease, are of the highest rank in selecting the remedy—a practical point it is well to remember. We should never neglect to inquire of a patient *whether any new symptoms have appeared* since the last visit or prescription and value any such highly.

Returning to the subject of indisposition: Having discovered such a case and determined that it does not require medication, the question arises, how is such a case to be managed? At first sight it would seem to be a very simple matter; merely to tell the patient bluntly that he does not need medicine, but only to mend his life and correct his habits according to the advice and instruction which you have given or will give. This view of the matter does not take into consideration the peculiarities of human nature as formed by ages and generations of habit and custom. Only occasionally do we meet a patient to whom we can give ideal advice and treatment. In spite of the rapid growth of the no-drug idea as promulgated by the various modern cults, the average patient *who goes to the doctor,* expects to get medicine. If he is so far advanced in his ideas as to believe in the no-drug theory he will probably not go to the doctor at all, but will seek out the osteopath or the Christian science healer. The patient who believes in drugs and goes to a doctor for treatment will be very likely to listen incredulously to your well-meant advice and will depart to tell his friends in anything but a respectful manner, that he thought you were a doctor, but he found that you were only a half-baked Christian scientist after all, or something to that effect. To direct his attention to his errors of living and order him to correct them is to apparently put the burden of cure upon him, and that is not what he wants at all. He expects us to bear that burden. That is what he comes to us for. Besides that, he often resents the assertion that his trouble is due to his own ignorance or wilfulness. There is a large class of people today—selfish, pleasure-seeking, luxury-loving, dissipating creatures, male and female—who demand of the physician relief from the pains and penalties of their hygienic sins, but are not willing to do their necessary part toward bringing this about. They want to "eat their cake and have it too."

We cannot afford to antagonize this class, either for their sakes or our own. We owe them a duty as well as ourselves, and few of us can afford to pick our patients. We must take them as they come and adjust ourselves to their individual needs and peculiarities. These in general are some of the cases which require tact in management. "You can catch more flies with molasses than with vinegar." We can gradually lead some of these people into better ways of life and thought and cure them of both their sickness and their sins, if we are patient and wise and tactful; while at the same time we are increasing the extent and influence of our practice. The physician who aims to be something more than a mere dispenser of palliatives, pills, and piffle, will never lack opportunities to magnify his profession and become a power for righteousness in his community, as well as a healer of its diseases. It is in dealing with such cases—the indispositions and habit disorders—that the *"second best remedy in the materia medica"* so often comes into use. Of course you all know what the second best remedy is. No? I am surprised that your education has been so neglected! But I am glad it is to be my privilege to teach you something you do not know. There are so few things that the average young doctor does not know!

In order to fully appreciate the value of the *second* best remedy, we must first clearly understand what is the *best* remedy in the materia medica. There cannot be any doubt in your minds as to that, I am sure. It is the *indicated remedy*. You also know that having once been found, the best remedy must be given *time to act,* and that its action must not be interfered with by other drugs or influences until it has accomplished all of which it is capable. You also know, or, if you do not, you will learn (if you keep your eyes open and your wits about you) that too many doses of the best remedy may spoil the case.

One of the distinguishing characteristics of a great painter is that he *knows when to stop.* Many a painting which would have been great, if the artist had known when to stop, has been weakened and spoiled by over-finishing. In his anxiety to perfect a few insignificant details he robs his work of its vitality—kills it. It is the same in treating a case. The problem is to give just enough medicine and not too much. Too many doses may spoil the case. I have referred to the class of people who expect and demand *medicine,* and are not satisfied unless they get it, until they have been taught better.

Now just here comes in the *second best remedy,* without which no good homœopathist could long practice medicine. Its technical name is *saccharum lactis officinalis;* abbreviated sac. lac. or s. l.; just plain sugar of milk! The young homœopath's best friend, the old doctor's reliance and a "very present help in time of trouble!"

The doctrine of *placebo,* from the Latin *placere,* to please; future, *placebo* "I shall please," is as old as medicine itself. Its psychological value is commensurate with the frailties and peculiarities of human nature. The traditional "breadpill" of our medical ancestors has given place, in the march of scientific progress, to the more elegant powder of virginal white, pure sugar of milk; or to the seductive little vial of sugar pills or tablets, artistically labeled and bestowed with impressive directions as to the exact number of pills for a dose and the precise hours of taking, with confident assurances of the happy effects to be expected, if directions are faithfully followed!

Marvelous are the results witnessed from the resort to this remedy in cases where it is indicated. I have seen it bring sleep to the "insomniac," when even morphine had failed. I have heard patients declare that it was the most effective cathartic they had ever taken and beg for a generous supply for future use; which supply I have usually refused on the ground that it was too powerful a remedy to be entrusted to the hands of the unskilled. It is indeed too powerful and too useful a remedy to be held lightly, or to be lightly used. The knowledge of its use is too dangerous to be disseminated among the laity. It should be as jealously guarded as a "trade-secret" worth millions. Never admit its use to any but the initiated, if you value your influence and reputation, but never fail to use it when your judgment dictates it.

Let us glance at a few of the practical uses of the placebo. You are called to a new case. You see the patient and make your examination. You decide that it is a case for medication. You have written down your symptom-findings and glanced over the record. The case is difficult and you are not able to decide offhand what remedy is indicated. You must have time and opportunity to study it up. The patient and friends want something done at once. Rapidly you run over the case in your mind. This patient is seriously ill. To make a mistake in the first prescription might be fatal, or it might prejudice the case by confusing it so that a quick and satisfactory cure would be impossible. Your reputation in the new family will depend upon your success. You must retain the confidence of the patient, but you must *have time and make no mistake.*

This is where your knowledge of the second best remedy comes into use. Calmly and confidently you prepare and administer a generous "s. l." powder, leave explicit directions for the use of as many subsequent doses as you deem judicious, make an appointment to see the patient again in an hour or two, or three, and then hie you to the seclusion of your library, where you proceed to apply your knowledge of how to study the case and find the remedy according to the principles of the Organon.

When you have worked out your case and found the remedy, you return. Then you enter the patient's presence as *master of the situation*—unless the Master of Destiny has ordained otherwise.

Does anybody consider that lost time? It is a pity that more time is not lost in that way! Thousands of cases might have been saved and many a professional reputation, by following such a course, instead of yielding to the silly panic-impulse to "do something quick," which almost invariably results in doing the wrong thing.

Patients do not usually die in a minute. There is always plenty of time to *do the right thing, always, at the right time.* If you *know* what the right thing is without reflection and study, do it at once. Give your remedy at once if you are sure of it, but not otherwise. If you are not sure, give sac. lac.

If the case is *really* pressing and demands immediate medication, retire to another room with your repertory then and there.

The very greatest of our prescribers—men like Bœnninghausen, Hering, Lippe, Wells, Biegler, of those who are gone, and almost all our expert prescribers of today, do not fail to carry their repertory with them to all cases, nor hesitate to use it in the presence of the patient if necessary. Instead of arousing distrust on the part of the patients, as you might think, it awakens confidence. To see a physician making a thorough examination, studying, "taking pains," showing a real interest in the case and a determination to do his best at the "psychological moment" (which is always the *present moment* with the man who is suffering), is calculated to inspire confidence at all times—except with fools, whom no physician wants for patients and who ought to be permitted to get off the earth as soon as possible for the benefit of posterity anyway.

Another use for the second best remedy is as a supplement to the indicated remedy. Experience shows that Hahnemann was right when he advised that *the remedy should be stopped as soon as signs of improvement appear,* and the curative reaction be allowed to go on without further repetition of doses as long as it will. This, of course, refers to the cases where repeated doses are given from the beginning. When improvement begins and you desire to cease medication, you will simply substitute sac. lac. for the remedy and watch your case.

The same course is pursued when treatment is begun with the *single dose,* by which method many of the most brilliant cures are made.

We may give enough sac. lac. powders to last during the interval between visits, or a vial of blank tablets or pellets; but be sure to moisten the tablets and pellets with alcohol, or put some unmedicated pellets in the sac. lac. powders. Patients have a way of investigating powders sometimes and counting the pellets. If they find no pellets they may become suspicious.

The medicine case should always contain a vial of blank pellets properly labeled for such use. One friend of mine always carries a duplicate case of vials containing blank pellets, but labeled as medicines to disarm suspicion.

These are some of the ways to use the second best remedy. If you follow the right course you will find more and more use for it, except with a few rare patients whom you can gradually educate up to the point where they come to realize that but little medicine and few doses are necessary, when a case is skillfully conducted. All this is quite in line with the most up-to-date teaching and thinking on therapeutic subjects. The use of placebo is simply one form, and a very powerful form of therapeutic suggestion; or, to use the still more recent term, psycho-therapy. In the habitual, systematic and judicious use of the harmless little powder of sac. lac. the homœopathist antedated all the modern cults of drugless healing, and even they have devised no more powerful nor efficient measure.

We are not under the necessity of sending our patients away, as Dr. Wm. Gilman Thompson, of Cornell University Medical College, had to do. He was holding a medical clinic before the senior class. To this clinic came a woman whose case was diagnosed as neurasthenia. Among the multitude of complaints she poured forth, she laid most stress upon *constipation;* but declared that she could and *would* not take any more cathartics.

Dr. Thompson pondered over the problem a few moments and then turned to the class and said: "Gentlemen, there is but one thing to do for this patient. We will send her to Boston. There, they will give her a *subconscious pill,* and she will get an *Immanuel Movement!"*

Many who are not susceptible to the "subconscious pill" will respond to the somewhat more tangible but none the less efficient sac. lac. powder, even among those who live in Boston!

Objection has been made to this mode of dealing with cases, by certain individuals with *very* delicate consciences, on the ground that it was not strictly honest! To practice even such a mild deception upon patients would violate their fine sense of honor! Besides, it tended to engender in patients a *habit* of dependence upon sac. lac., and to demoralize the physician who followed the practice!

Recall the words of HIM who said: "Woe unto you, Scribes and Pharisees, hypocrites! for ye pay tithes of mint and anise and cummin, and have omitted the *weightier matters of the law,* judgment, mercy and faith; these ought ye to have done, and not to leave the other undone. Ye blind guides which strain at a gnat and swallow a camel!"

He who said that, anointed the eyes of a blind man with "clay mixed with spittle," bade him go and wash in the pool of Siloam, and he recovered his sight—healed by *faith;* awakened by the therapeutic suggestion of a *clay placebo* and an order to take a bath!

Any harmless measure which tends to arouse the curative reaction of the organism through the awakening of faith and confident expectation, is not only right but legitimate and sometimes indispensable.

But what shall we say of the men who have been so pained at the thought of using the placebo, when we find them violating every fundamental law and principle of the art whose name they profess before the world, by using powerful drugs in such a manner in their treatment of the sick, in both public and private practice, as to do irreparable injury?

Or what shall we say of men prominently before the public as official representatives of homœopathy in colleges and hospital, who herd patients in a Metropolitan Hospital ward, arbitrarily denominate them a "class," without regard to their individual symptoms, and give them all, indiscriminately, hypodermic injections of "a preparation of digitalis" for their hearts?

This is indeed neglecting *"the weightier matters of the law."* It is the irony of fate that makes it possible to say such a thing of men who conduct a great hospital which was specifically founded and financed for the purpose of dispensing the blessings of homœopathy to the poor of the great city.

And what about the young men who have come from far and wide to the colleges connected with such hospitals, and pay their money in good faith for such instruction in the methods and principles of homœopathy, who are called upon to witness such perversions of all true therapeutic principles, to say nothing of homœopathy? Should they not be considered?

President Cleveland immortalized himself by declaring that "Public Office Is a Public Trust."

President Roosevelt endeared himself to the people, and will go down in history as the great exponent of "The Square Deal."

These two great leaders, each in his own way, have thus voiced the principles of *common honesty* in the conduct of public and private affairs. The people have listened and responded. The world is waking up, for, as President Lincoln said: "You can fool some of the people all of the time; you can fool all of the people some of the time, but you cannot fool all the people all of the time."

When homœopathic colleges teach homœopathy in every appropriate chair; when homœopathic hospitals and homœopathic clinics are conducted on homœopathic principles; and when homœopathic physicians make at least a sincere *attempt* to prescribe homœopathic remedies for their patients; then, and not before, will the principles of *common honesty* find their application in the homœopathic medical profession.

It is a breach of trust to do otherwise. The *moral obligation* is upon every man who is affiliated with a homœopathic institution, and upon every physician who professes the name of homœopathy, to be true to homœopathic principles.

It is not many years since the late Judge Barrett, of the Supreme Court, in a decision which he handed down in a certain case, declared that the *legal obligation* rested upon every professedly homœopathic physician to practice according to homœopathic principles; and that he was liable at law if he did not do so. The people who give their money to found and sustain homœopathic institutions have some right in this matter which should be respected.

We have now a "pure food law" which requires that all goods shall be "true to label." The time may come, and perhaps is not far distant, when we shall have a "pure practice law," which will require that a man who represents himself as a graduate of a homœopathic school and a practitioner of homœopathy, shall be required to practice in accordance with the principles of that school or suffer the penalty of his misrepresentation—in other words, that *he* shall be "true to label." He will not be able in that day, as he is now, to advertise, '57 varieties!" There is but *one* variety of homœopathy, and that is the homœopathy of Hahnemann, the principles of which are plainly laid down in the Organon. All other varieties are fraudulent, concocted of impure materials and injurious to health, like the inferior canned goods of the manufacturers, which they try to preserve with antiseptics. If some of the fraudulent homœopaths were compelled, like the food manufacturers, to state on their labels the names and percentages of the foreign ingredients in their wares, it might be better for the people, but they would have to enlarge either their labels or their packages in order to make room for the list.

With all this there is no need to be pessimistic. The leaders of the homœopathic profession are awake to the true state of affairs. They are demanding of their colleges and teachers that homœopathic principles shall be taught, and the colleges are responding as rapidly as they can, hampered as they are by the presence of some men in their faculties who are antagonistic to everything homœopathic. They recognize that the future of homœopathy depends upon the *young men* who are coming up; upon the classes now within college halls; that the long neglected principles and methods of homœopathy must be restored to their true place in the college curriculum and taught by men who love the art of healing and are imbued with the *spirit* of homœopathy and the love of it! We may know the principles—the *science* of homœopathy—but unless we love the *art,* and practice it, we will fail in the highest department of our calling. Never was there such need as there is today for pure homœopathy, nor such opportunities for young men of enthusiasm and earnest purpose, who are thoroughly trained in homœopathic methods. The colleges need them as teachers. The hospitals need them as internes and visitors, and in other official positions. The people need them as practical healers. Prepared for *that* work, *"The world is our oyster."*

CHAPTER XI

Symptomatology

The Homœopathic Materia Medica.—The Materia Medica of Hahnemann is an enduring monument to the genius of its author, original in its conception and design and unique in its form and contents. Its foundation is on the bedrock of natural law. It is constructed of the cut stones of accurately observed facts, laid up in the cement of irrefragible logic. Over its portals are graven the words, *Similia Similibus Curantur; Simplex, Simile, Minimum.*

Hahnemann, on apprehending a new general principle in therapeutics, was confronted with the problem of creating an entirely new materia medica by means of which the principle might be applied in practice. If diseases were to be treated according to the principle of symptom-similarity it was necessary to know what symptoms drugs would produce in healthy persons, since these would be the only symptoms which could possibly resemble the symptoms of sick persons. There was no materia medica in existence which contained the facts or phenomena of the action of drugs upon the healthy. The existent materia medicas contained only the incidental observations, theories and opinions of drug action of men who gave drugs to the sick or treated cases of poisoning upon purely empirical and speculative assumptions; and these were given, not singly, but in such combination and mixtures as to render impossible any intelligent conception of what the action of a single drug might be.

Undismayed by the magnitude of the task, Hahnemann set about creating a materia medica which should embody the facts of drug action upon the healthy. He instituted "provings" of drugs upon himself, members of his family, friends, students and fellow practitioners, keeping all under the most rigid scrutiny and control, and carefully recording every fact and the conditions under which it was elicited. This work was continued for many years, parts of it being published from time to time, until the mass of material had reached enormous proportions.

Adopting the plan of arranging the drug symptoms thus derived according to the anatomical parts and regions of the body in which they occurred, as the most rational and simple method of classification for the purpose of comparison with disease symptoms, Hahnemann constructed and published, first, the Materia Medica Pura, and later, The Chronic Diseases, the greater part of which is composed of provings of drugs. Covering nearly three thousand royal octavo pages, they constitute one of the most stupendous works of original experimentation and research ever attempted and carried out by one man. To this original work of Hahnemann many and large additions have been made by later workers.

The vast collection of symptoms of which the materia medica of Homœopathy is composed is incomprehensible without an understanding of the principles upon which it is based. In a good working homœopathic library there are about two hundred volumes, by many authors, upon the subject of materia medica, including special collections and classifications, repertories, charts and indexes of symptoms. Confronted by such a mass of material it is no wonder that the student is at first confused and discouraged. But when the basic principle has been explained to him and he has learned the meaning of symptoms, their method of classification and interpretation, and when he has seen the means of ready reference provided, his bewilderment gives way to admiration.

The task of mastering the materia medica, vast and even impossible as it seems, is comparatively simple. The compass that points the way through the seeming wilderness of symptoms is the principle of *Similia*—the remedial law of homœopathy.

When the drug symptoms recorded in the homœopathic materia medica are seen to be exact counterparts of the symptoms of disease, and it is explained that medicines cure disease by virtue of this similarity of symptoms, the reason for the existence of the materia medica in its characteristic form is evident. *The arrangement of symptoms according to an anatomical scheme is for the purpose of comparison—symptoms of drugs with the symp-*

toms of disease. Given the basic principle and its corollaries, the rest is merely a matter of mastering the logical classification and interpretation of symptoms and the use of the manuals, indexes and repertories provided.

Symptomatology.—The first requisite to a correct understanding of the subject of symptomatology is to know the full meaning of the word "symptom" and all that it involves.

Knowledge of the true nature and constitution of a symptom is necessary in proving or testing medicines; in the examination of a patient; in the study of the materia medica and in the selection and management of the indicated remedy. It is a standard by which to judge the reliability of a proving, a clinical case, an examination record, or the professions of a newcoming *confrere*.

Ignorance of the nature and constitution of symptoms on the part of provers, directors of provings and physicians has resulted in the production of certain provings and books on materia medica which are practically worthless, and the publication of reports of cases which have served no better purpose than to float their authors' names on the sea of printer's ink. Such productions, consisting largely of commonplace generalities, indefinite pathological names and pseudo-scientific instrumental and laboratory findings, reveal the ignorance of their authors of all that goes into the making of reliable cures and provings conducted under classic homœopathic principles. The result is useless to the prescriber because it does not contain the elements upon which a homœopathic prescription can be based.

It is not intended to belittle or ridicule laboratory and instrumental findings. Such observations are useful and necessary for certain scientific, particularly diagnostic and pathological purposes; but they are only a part, and a very small part of homœopathic provings, or of clinical symptom-records designed for the use of the prescriber. They cannot take the place of the more important things which have been left out. What those things are will appear as the definition of symptoms proceeds.

Symptoms Defined.—In general, a symptom is any evidence of disease, or change from a state of health. In materia medica no relevant fact is too insignificant to be overlooked. There is a place and use for every fact, for science has learned that "Nature never trifles." A symptom which appears trifling to the careless or superficial examiner may become, in the hands of the expert, the key which unlocks a difficult problem in therapeutics.

Hahnemann defines symptoms broadly as, "any manifestation of a deviation from a former state of health, perceptible by the patient, the individuals around him, or the physician." We have here the basis of the common division of symptoms into two general classes—Subjective and Objective.

Hahnemann further defines symptoms as "evidences of the operation of the influences which disturb the harmonious play of the functions, the vital principle as a spiritual-dynamis." (Substantial, entitative source of vital power and activity.)

Subjective Symptoms.—Subjective Symptoms are symptoms which are discoverable by the patient alone, such as pain and other morbid sensations of body or mind, presenting no external indications. With Hahnemann's announcement of the doctrine of the Totality of the Symptoms as the basis of the homœopathic prescription, it became possible for the first time in the history of medicine to utilize all the phenomena of disease. Prior to Hahnemann's time two of the most frequently occurring and important groups of symptoms were practically ignored—the mental symptoms and the subjective symptoms. The "regular" practitioner of medicine even today is interested very little in subjective symptoms. They play but a very small part in governing the practical treatment of his case. To him they are merely inarticulate cries of suffering, serving only to suggest the direction in which investigations are to be made by physical and laboratory methods for discovering the supposed tangible cause of the disease, and the location and character of its lesions.

Under the new system of therapeutics devised by Hahnemann subjective symptoms naturally took their proper place in the study of the case. As expressions of the interior states of the organism, and particularly of the psychic and mental states, they take the highest rank. Nothing can supersede them. They constitute the only direct avenue of approach to that inner sphere which must otherwise remain closed to our investigation, except as it is indirectly revealed in certain automatic or involuntary objective symptoms from which more or less accurate deductions can sometimes be made. They enable the physician to view disease from the standpoint of the patient. How great an advantage they afford to the prescriber can be appreciated only when we are deprived of them, as in the case of infants and animals, and find how much more difficult is our task under such circumstances.

Before Hahnemann's genius opened up the new way pain was merely pain. To discriminate between various kinds of pain; to analyze and classify pains, and not only pains, but all other subjective sensations and feelings, and to relate them as phenomena of disease to remedies, as Hahnemann did, had never been thought of before. It is ridiculed and scoffed at today by those who do not see that there is something radically wrong with a system of medicine that practically ignores the great bulk of the symptoms of almost every case and tantalizes the patient by learned explanations of their cause; by assurances that they are of no consequence; or, if his clamor becomes too loud, clubs him into silence with an opiate.

Objective Symptoms.—Hahnemann defines objective symptoms as, "the expression of disease in the sensations and functions of that side of the organism exposed to the senses of the physician and bystanders." In this peculiar definition there is an allusion to his definition of disease as a dynamical disturbance of the vital force and of Medicine as, "a pure science of experience, which can and must rest on clear facts and sensible phenomena clearly cognizable by the senses." There is also a reminder that there is more in an objective symptom than is perceptible to the eye alone. The subjective "sensations and functions" of the visibly affected organ or part are to be considered as well as the purely objective signs. Hahnemann here implies that functional and sensational disturbances precede organic changes; and this is consistent with his basic premise that all disease is primarily a dynamical disturbance of the life principle. He never loses sight of this fundamental conception of the nature of disease.

Totality of the Symptoms.—"Totality of the Symptoms" is an expression peculiar to homœopathy which requires special attention. It is highly important to understand exactly what it means and involves, because the totality of the symptoms is the true and only basis for every homœopathic prescription.

Hahnemann (Org., Par. 6) says:—"The ensemble or totality of these available signs or symptoms, represents in its full extent the disease itself; that is, they constitute the true and only form of which the mind is capable of conceiving." The expression has a two-fold meaning. It represents the disease and it also represents the remedy, as language represents thought.

1. The Totality of the Symptoms means, first, the totality of each individual symptom.

A single symptom is more than a single fact; it is a fact, with its history, its origin, its location, its progress or direction, and its conditions.

Every complete symptom has three essential elements:—Location, Sensation and Modality.

By *location* is meant the part, organ, tissue or function of body or mind in which the symptom appears.

By *sensation* is meant the impression, or consciousness of an impression upon the central system through the medium of the sensory or afferent nerves, or through one of the organs of senses; a feeling, or state of consciousness produced by an external stimulus, or by some change in the internal state of the body. A sensation may also be a purely mental or physical reaction, such as fright, fear, anger, grief or jealousy.

By *modality* we refer to the circumstances and conditions that affect or modify a symptom, of which the conditions of aggravation and amelioration are the most important. Dr. William Boericke well said:

"The modalities of a drug are the pathognomonic symptoms of the Materia Medica."

By *"aggravation"* is meant an increase or intensification of already existing symptoms by some appreciable circumstance or condition.

"Aggravation" is also used in homœopathic parlance to describe those conditions in which, under the action of a deeply acting homœopathic medicine (or from other causes), latent disease becomes active and expresses itself in the return of the old symptoms or the appearance of new symptoms. In such cases it represents the reaction of the organism to the stimulus of a well selected medicine, and is generally curative in its nature.

"*Amelioration*" is technically used to express the modification of relief, or diminution of intensity in any of the symptoms, or in the state of the patient as a whole, by medication, or by the influence of any agency, circumstance or condition.

2. The Totality of the Symptoms means *all the symptoms of the case which are capable of being logically combined into a harmonious and consistent whole, having form, coherency and individuality.* Technically, the totality is more (and may be less) than the mere numerical totality of the symptoms. It includes the "*concomitance*" or form in which symptoms are grouped.

Hahnemann (Org., Par. 7) calls the totality, "*this image (or picture) reflecting outwardly the internal essence of the disease, i. e., of the suffering life force.*"

The word used is significant and suggestive. A picture is a *work of art,* which appeals to our esthetic sense as well as to our intellect. Its elements are form, color, light, shade, tone, harmony, and perspective. As a composition it *expresses an idea,* it may be of sentiment or fact; but it does this by the harmonious combination of its elements into a whole—a totality. In a well balanced picture each element is given its full value and its right relation to all the other elements.

So it is in the symptom picture which is technically called the Totality. *The totality must express an idea.* When studying a case from the diagnostic standpoint, for example, certain symptoms are selected as having a known pathological relation to each other, and upon these is based the diagnosis. The classification of symptoms thus made represents the *diagnostic idea.* Just so the "totality of the symptoms," considered as the basis of a homœopathic prescription, represents the *therapeutic idea.* These two groups may be and often are different. The elements which go to make up the *therapeutic totality* must be as definitely and logically related and consistent as are the elements which go to make up the *diagnostic totality.*

The "totality" is not, therefore, a mere haphazard, fortuitous jumble of symptoms thrown together without rhyme or reason, any more than a similar haphazard collection of pathogenetic symptoms in a proving constitutes Materia Medica.

The Totality means the *sum of the aggregate of the symp-*

toms: Not merely the numerical aggregate—the entire number of the symptoms as particulars or single symptoms—but their sum total, their organic whole as an individuality. As a machine set up complete and in perfect working order is more than a numerical aggregate of its single dissociated parts, so the Totality is more than the mere aggregate of its constituent symptoms. It is the numerical aggregate *plus the idea or plan which unites them in a special manner to give them its characteristic form.* As the parts of a machine cannot be thrown together in any haphazard manner, but each part must be fitted to each other part in a certain definite relation according to the preconceived plan or design—"assembled," as the mechanics say—so the symptoms of a case must be "assembled" in such a manner that they constitute an identity, an individuality, which may be seen and recognized as we recognize the personality of a friend.

The same idea underlies the phrase, *"Genius of the Remedy."* Genius, in this sense, being the dominant influence, or the essential principle of the remedy which gives it its individuality.

The idea of the Totality as an abstract form, or figure, has been applied to the materia medica as a whole. The materia medica as a whole is the sum total of the symptoms of all proved medicines—a grand, all inclusive figure which may be imagined or personified in the form of a human being or "super-man," this conception being based upon the anatomical, physiological and psychological plan or framework of the materia medica.

The idea is applicable in exactly the same way in pathology. Disease in general, considered as a whole, is composed of the totality of all the symptoms which represent it to our senses. The pathological totality, also, can be personified or pictured by the imagination in the form of a human being.

Starting with this conception some of our ingenious writers have amused themselves and added to the gaiety of the profession by personifying medicines, microbes and maladies and casting them in all sorts of roles—a dramatic whimsy which has its value as an educational expedient for a certain type of mind.

The materia medica from this point of view becomes a portrait gallery of diseases, a sort of medical "Rogues Gallery" by means of which we may identify the thieves who steal away our health and comfort and bring them to justice. In homœopathic practice, to carry out the simile, we merely "set a thief to catch a thief."

As a constructive principle, therefore, the idea of the Totality enters into the formation not only of the materia medica as a whole, but of every remedy and every symptom.

Each disease, each individual case of disease and each symptom of disease has its totality or individual form.

If the "day books" or records of a good proving are examined it will be seen that the symptoms of each prover are set down chronologically in the order of their occurrence; that each symptom is as complete as possible in its elements of locality, sensation and modality; that the symptoms are stated mostly in the vernacular, the plain simple language of the layman, who describes phenomena as they appear to him, simply, graphically, or by analogy or homely comparison. The record of these facts with the remarks and observations of the director of the proving constitutes a "proving," in which exists the elements from which the Materia Medica is constructed.

The Day Books of the provers are not the Materia Medica. Not until this mass of material has been analyzed, sifted, classified according to its anatomical, physiological and pathological relations and had its general and particular characteristics logically deduced, does it become materia medica for practical use. Many things in a proving must be interpreted in the light of anatomy, physiology, pathology, or psychology before they are available for therapeutic use, just as the statements of a patient in regard to his sufferings must be interpreted in making a diagnosis or in making a prescription.

The true Totality, therefore, is a Work of Art, formed by the mind of the artist from the crude materials at his command, which are derived from a proving or from a clinical examination of the patient.

It is important that these points should be understood, because, otherwise, there is liability to err in several directions.

1. Error may arise in placing too much emphasis upon a single symptom, or perhaps actually prescribing on a single symptom as many thoughtlessly do.

2. Error may arise in attempting to fit a remedy to a mass of indefinite, unrelated or fragmentary symptoms by a mechanical comparison of symptom with symptom, by which the prescriber becomes a mere superficial "symptom coverer."

3. Failing in both these ways the prescriber may fall to the level of the so-called "pathological prescribers," who empirically base their treatment upon a theoretical pathological diagnosis and end in prescribing unnecessary and injurious sedatives, stimulants, combination tablets, and other crude mixtures of common practice.

The physician who knows what a symptom is from the homœopathic standpoint and how to elicit it; who knows what the totality of the symptoms means and how to construct it, and who has the intelligence, the patience and the honesty to study his case until he finds it will not be guilty of such practice.

Characteristics and Keynotes.—In paragraph 153 of The Organon, Hahnemann says that in comparing the collective symptoms of the natural disease with drug symptoms for the purpose of finding the specific curative remedy, "the more striking, singular, uncommon and peculiar (*characteristic*) signs and symptoms of the case are *chiefly and almost solely* to be kept in view; for it is more particularly these that very similar ones in the list of symptoms of the selected medicine must correspond to, in order to constitute it the most suitable for effecting the cure. The more general (common) and undefined symptoms; loss of appetite, headache, debility, etc., demand but little attention when of that vague and indefinite character, if they cannot be more accurately described, as symptoms of such a general nature are observed in almost every disease and drug."

This seems a sufficiently clear description of what Hahnemann meant by "characteristic" symptoms; and yet the term has been the subject of much discussion and many have differed as to what constitutes a "characteristic."

Confusion arose and still exists through the inability on the part of many to reconcile the teaching of this paragraph with the apparently conflicting doctrine of The Totality of the Symptoms as the only basis of a true homœopathic prescription. These have taken refuge either in the mechanical "symptom covering" already referred to, as fulfilling their conception of the "totality;" or in what is knows as "keynote prescribing," which, as they practice it, means prescribing on some single symptom which they (perhaps whimsically) regard as the "keynote" of the case.

The fundamental mistake here has been in the failure to distinguish between the *numerical totality* and the *related* or *logical totality*, as already explained.

Both of these misapprehensions should be recognized and corrected.

The real "keynote system," as taught and practiced by the late Dr. Henry N. Guernsey (but perverted by many) does not conflict with the doctrine of the totality of the symptoms, nor does it fall short of complying with Hahnemann's injunction to pay most attention to the peculiar and characteristic symptoms of the case. It is, in fact, strictly Hahnemannian. The truth is that Dr. Guernsey simply invented a new name for the old Hahnemannian idea.

A synopsis of Dr. Guernsey's keynote method will be of value in this connection.

The term "keynote" is merely suggestive as used in this connection. the reference being to the analogy between materia medica and music. This analogy is shown in the use of other musical terms in medicine, as when the patient speaks of being "out of tune," or the physician speaks of the "tone" of the organism. Disease is correctly defined as a loss of *harmony* in function and sensation.

The keynote in music is defined as "the fundamental note or tone of which the whole piece is accommodated." In pathology the term "pathognomonic symptom" expresses what might be called the keynote of the disease, or that which differentiates it from other diseases of a similar character.

In comparing the symptoms of medicines we find that each medicine presents peculiar differences from all other medicine. These differences by which one remedy is distinguished from another, are the "keynotes" of the remedy, according to Dr. Guernsey.

It does not mean that the keynote of the case alone is to be met by the keynote of the remedy alone and that the other features of the case or remedy are to be ignored. The keynote is simply the predominating symptom or feature which directs attention to the totality. Its function is merely suggestive. A prescription is not based upon a keynote, considered as one symptom, no matter how "peculiar" it may seem. Its utility lies in this: that when the prescriber has become familiar with these "keynotes" or "characteristics" of remedies he will be able more quickly to find the remedy in a given case because the field of selection has been narrowed. When he recognizes such a keynote in the symptoms of a case it suggests or recalls to mind a medicine, or medicines, having a similar keynote. Reference to the repertory and materia medica will verify and complete the comparison. There is usually something peculiar in the case, some prominent feature or striking combination of symptoms that directs the attention to a certain drug, and this is what Dr. Guernsey called a keynote.

The misunderstanding and abuse of this method has caused it to fall somewhat into discredit. But considering Guernsey's "keynotes" and Hahnemann's "characteristics" as synonymous terms, which they are, and making legitimate use of Guernsey's method, it has value.

A characteristic or keynote symptom is a generalization drawn from the particular symptoms by logical deduction. Evidently the characteristic or peculiar symptoms of a case cannot be determined until a complete examination has elicited *all the symptoms of the case* (the numerical totality) for purposes of comparison. This having been done there are various ways of selecting the characteristics.

Dr. Adolph Lippe illustrated his method in this way: "In many cases," he says, "the characteristic symptoms will consist in the result obtained by deducting all the symptoms generally pertaining *to the disease* with which the patient suffers, from those elicited by a thorough examination *of the case.*" In other words *the characteristic symptoms are the symptoms peculiar to the individual patient, rather than the symptoms common to the disease.*

He illustrated this by a case, as follows: "The patient was attacked by cholera. All the characteristic symptoms of cholera were present; but in this individual case there was (1) an unusual noise in the intestines, as if a fluid were being emptied out of a bottle. (2) The discharge came away *with a gush.* Of what pathological value these symptoms were we know not. Still they formed part of the totality which we must cover. Deducting from the (numerical) totality of the symptoms those common to the disease, we were in possession of the characteristic symptoms of the patient.

"We found that those two symptoms are also characteristic of *Jatropha curcas,* and that this remedy, at the same time, has caused symptoms corresponding with the general pathological condition." Jatropha promptly cured the case.

The selection of a curative remedy in this case, therefore, was governed by two symptoms of no known pathological value, and of seemingly trifling character. Yet these two symptoms were what gave the case its individuality, and unerringly pointed out the curative remedy.

This case is a beautiful example of the kind of work for which Dr. Lippe was famous. It illustrates the necessity of being familiar with the natural history, symptomatology and diagnosis of disease. Dr. Lippe could not have decided that these two symptoms were peculiar and characteristic if he had been unfamiliar with the symptoms of cholera. Neither could he have selected these two symptoms as peculiar if he had not had the rest of the symptoms before him for comparison. The mistake of arbitrarily picking out some "freak" symptom, and giving a remedy which has a corresponding symptom, should be avoided. Dr. Guernsey did not teach prescribing on a single symptom.

In the preface to the first edition of his great work on obstetrics Dr. Guernsey presents the subject of "keynote prescribing" in another way. He says: "The plan of treatment may seem to some rather novel, and perhaps on its first view, objectionable, *inasmuch as it may seem like prescribing for single symptoms, whereas such is not the fact.* It is only meant to state some strong characteristic symptom, which will often be found the governing symptom, and on referring to the Symptomen Codex or Materia Medica all the others will be there if this one is.

"There must be a head to everything; so in symptomatology; if the most interior or peculiar symptom, or keynote, is discernible, it will (usually) be found that all the other symptoms of the case will be also found under that remedy which produces this peculiar one, if the remedy be well proven. It will be necessary, in order to prescribe efficiently, to discover in every case that which characterizes one remedy above another in every combination of symptoms that exist. There is certainly that in every case of illness which pre-eminently characterizes that case, or causes it to differ from every other. So in the remedy to be selected, there is and must be a peculiar *combination of symptoms,* a characteristic or keynote. Strike that and all the others are easily touched, attuned or sounded. There is only one keynote to any piece of music, however complicated, and that note governs all the others in the various parts, no matter how many variations, trills, accompaniments, etc."

If it is understood that the "keynote" to a case may and often does exist in, or consist of, a "peculiar combination," as Dr. Guernsey puts it, and that it is not merely some peculiar, single, possibly incomplete symptom which the tyro is always mistakenly looking for, the subject is cleared of part of its obscurity. Dr. Guernsey might have summed up the whole matter in one word—Generalization, which has been discussed at length in the chapters on the logic of homœopathy.

Dr. Lippe, discussing characteristic symptoms, wrote as follows: "When medicines are submitted to provings upon the healthy they develop a variety of symptoms in a variety of provers. Each prover has his own peculiar, characteristic individuality affected by the medicine in a peculiar manner; other differently constituted individuals experience different, yet similar, peculiar symptoms from the same medicine. There is a similarity and a difference evident upon close comparison. In like manner diseases and all other external influences affect different individualities differently, yet similarly. The physiological school and its followers accept in disease only what is general (common) to all those affected by it; in medicinal provings in the same manner they accept only that which has been experienced alike by many. In both cases they simply (sic) generalize. The homœopathic school reverses this order. Accepting all the symptoms experienced by the differently constituted provers, they consider as peculiarly characteristic the individual symptoms of the patient; those *not* generally experienced by others suffering from a similar form of disease."

This is individualizing with a vengeance! In aspersing the process of what he calls generalizing Dr. Lippe traduces the very instrument he is apparently unconsciously using, but misusing the word. One is the traditional pathological-diagnostic method based upon an arbitrary and artificial classification of only the common or gross phenomena of disease; the other is the homœopathic natural or inductive method of modern science, based upon *all* the phenomena of the case, but paying particular attention to the *uncommon* and peculiar features, never forgetting that we always have an *individual patient* to treat and cure.

Dr. P. P. Wells says: "Characteristic symptoms are *those which individualize both the disease and the drug.* That which distinguishes the individual case of disease to be treated from other members of its class is to find its resemblance among those effects of the drug which distinguish it from other drugs. This is what we mean when we say that with these the law of cure has chiefly to do. When we say 'like cures like' this is the 'like' we mean."

Characteristics may sometimes be symptoms observed only as a result of the closest scrutiny, like the apparently trifling clues in a mysterious murder case which the ordinary detective overlooks or ignores, but which a Sherlock Holmes pounces upon and utilizes with amazing logical acumen to clear up what is otherwise impossible of solution. Their value depends upon who is using them. An Agassiz or a Leidy, placed in possession of a fragment of bone, or the scale of a fish, found in the remains of some pre-glacial geologic period, will reconstruct for us not only the animal or fish from which it came, but unfold a whole chapter of natural history, picture the scene and repeople a forgotten period of earth's history before our delighted eyes.

Dr. Charles G. Raue pointed out that scarcely one of the "keynotes" or characteristic symptoms belongs exclusively to a single remedy, and cautioned us not to diagnose a remedy on one symptom only, be it ever so characteristic. "While in some cases," he says, "it may point exactly to the remedy, it cannot do so in every case, as it is not rational to suppose that the whole sphere of action of a remedy, which is often extensive and complex, should find its unerring expression and indication in one symptom. But such characteristics are of great aid in the selection of the remedy, as they define the circle of remedies out of which we must select."

Dr. Hering, in his quaint fashion, years before the "keynote system" was ever heard of, said: "Every stool must have at least three legs, if it is to stand alone." He advised selecting at least three characteristic symptoms as the basis of prescribing.

A milking stool will stand upon one leg—*if you sit on it* and thus provide your own two legs as the other necessary props; but even then, as every farmer's boy knows by bitter experience, a vicious kick, or a "corkscrew swat" from the old cow's tail may upset the youthful milker and his pail of milk and bring him to grief.

So it is wise to always give the symptomatic milk-stool as broad a base and as many legs as possible. The youthful prescriber will get many a vicious kick from refractory cases. He may be knocked sprawling and lose his pail of milk a few times, but he will be able to avoid this when he has learned the peculiarities of his patient as well as I learned the peculiarities of my bovine kicker when I was a boy.

The Totality is an ideal not always to be realized. As a matter of fact, in practical experience, it is often impossible to complete every symptom, or even a large part of the symptoms. Patients have not observed, or cannot state all these points. They will give fragments; the location of a sensation which they cannot describe, or a sensation which they cannot locate; or they will give a sensation, properly located, but without being able, through ignorance, stupidity, failure to observe or forgetfulness, to state the conditions of time and circumstances under which it appeared. Sometimes no amount of questioning will succeed in bringing out the missing elements of some of the symptoms.

What is to be done under such circumstances? Make a guess at the remedy? Give two or three remedies, in alternation? Give a combination tablet? Or "dope" the patient with quinine or morphine? Rather than do any of these things, follow the advice of my old preceptor, Dr. P. P. Wells. Sometimes, when I approached him with a difficult case, he would assume a quizzical expression and ask, "Don't you know what to do?" On being answered in the negative he would say, "If you don't know what to do, do *nothing*—until you *do* know;" emphasizing the injunction with a characteristic downward stroke of his right forefinger. Then he would go over the case and show what should be done and how to do it.

It was he who taught me Boenninghausen's method of dealing with such cases. And I thought the more of it because he had known Boenninghausen and had received instruction and treatment from the Grand Old Man personally, while traveling in Europe.

Boenninghausen's Therapeutic Pocketbook.—Boenninghausen's famous Therapeutic Pocketbook was devised primarily to deal with just such cases. The materia medica contains a great number of incomplete symptoms. Until Boenninghausen's time this constituted one of the greatest obstacles to successful homœopathic prescribing. Boenninghausen first conceived the idea of completing these symptoms partly by analogy, and partly by clinical observation of curative effects. He discovered that many if not all of *the modalities* of a case were *general in their relation,* and were not necessarily confined to the particular symptoms with which they had first been observed. The "aggravation in a warm room" of Pulsatilla, for example, might first have been observed as applying to a headache. Boenninghausen assumed that this modality applied to *all* the symptoms—*to the patient himself,* in other words; and that this modality, once discovered in relation to any particular symptom of Pulsatilla, might be used to complete all other symptoms of Pulsatilla which, up to that time, had been incomplete in respect to their modalities. Experience proved this to be true.

Out of this grew the idea that all other combinations of symptoms might be thus made. By classifying the characteristic features of medicines in certain general relations to each other, in such a way that one part could be used to complete another, the prescriber might always be able to construct a related totality, even with apparently fragmentary symptoms.

Starting with the basic idea that every symptom is composed of the three elements of locality, sensation and modality, and that fragmentary symptoms may be completed by analogy or by supplementary clinical observation of the curative effects of similar remedies, Boenninghausen, in his Therapeutic Pocketbook, distributes the elements of all symptoms, pathogenetic and clinical, according to this analysis, into seven distinct parts or sections which, taken together, form a grand totality. (1) Moral and Intellectual Faculties; (2) Locality or Seat of the Symptoms; (3) Morbid Conditions and Sensations; (4) Sleep and Dreams; (5) Circulation and Fever; (6) Modalities, Etiology, etc.; (7) Concordances. Each of these sections is subdivided into rubrics containing the names of remedies arranged alphabetically under the symptoms to which they correspond.

Of this arrangement he says: "Although each part ought to be considered as a complete whole, it never yields, however, more than a part of a symptom, which receives its complement from one or many of the other parts. In odontalgia, for example, the seat of the pain is found in the second, the nature of the pain in the third, the exacerbation or diminution of pain, according to time, place, or circumstance in the sixth; and that which is necessary as an accessory to complete the description of the malady, and warrant the choice of medicines, must be sought in the different chapters."

By this method, as Dr. Wm. Boericke observes: "a remedy is selected for a case that is found to possess in its symptomatology marked action (1) in a certain location, (2) to correspond with the sensation, and (3) to possess the modality; *without necessarily having in the proving the very symptom resulting from the combination.* It is to be inferred that a *full* proving *would* have it, however. For instance, a patient with a tearing pain in the left hip, relieved by motion, greatly worse in the afternoon, would receive Lycopodium, not because Lycopodium has so far produced in the healthy such a symptom, but because from the study of its symptoms as recorded in the materia medica, we do find that it effects the left hip prominently (locality); that its pain in various parts of the body are 'tearing' (sensation); and that its general symptoms are relieved by motion and aggravated in the afternoon (modality)."

The experience of nearly a century has verified the truth of Boenninghausen's idea and enabled us, in the use of his masterpiece, The Therapeutic Pocketbook, to overcome to a great extent the imperfections and limitations of our materia medica.

In constructing a materia medica from the materials of the provings, all the symptoms of the different provers of the same drug are collected under the name of the drug. The second step is to distribute the symptoms thus collected under the names of the various parts, organs and functions of the body affected by the drug. This localizes the phenomena of each drug and gives the materia medica its anatomical and physiological structure.

When all the symptoms have been collected and arranged in this form under the name of the medicine, it represents a sick man, whose likeness may be met almost any day in the actual world. The drug symptoms are in fact disease symptoms, artificially induced. In other words they are symptoms of a drug disease. The significant thing is that drug diseases or poisonings accidentally or intentionally produced, *are similar to natural diseases*—so similar that it is sometimes difficult to distinguish them. A person poisoned to a certain degree by arsenic, or camphor, or veratrum album, for example, presents an appearance so similar to one suffering from cholera, that any one but an expert might be deceived. If this is so strikingly true of the gross and violent phenomena produced by poisonings, it is equally true of the milder, finer and less obvious symptoms which result from proving drugs in small or moderate doses.

Language of the Materia Medica.—The symptoms of the homœopathic materia medica, experienced by the provers, are expressed in plain and common terms. The language of everyday life is used, not the technical language of the medical profession. For this reason, the homœopathic materia medica is enduring. It is not subject to the influence of the transitory theories of general medicine, with its constantly changing terminology and bewildering array of newly invented names. So long as common language endures, the homœopathic materia medica will be intelligible and useful to every person who can read and write.

It is enduring also because it is a record of the facts of actual, voluntary experience, in a sphere and under conditions open and common to all men. In other words, the "experiments" of homœopathy are made by men, upon men, for men under the *natural* conditions which belong to the everyday life of all men. They are not necessarily conducted in elaborately equipped technical laboratories, nor by using and abusing poor, dumb animals, "whose only language is a cry," who are often forced to give up their lives, under unspeakable torture, to bolster up the theory, or satisfy the curiosity of some cold-blooded man of science. While knowledge gained by vivisection may be valuable to the surgeon, it is unnecessary for the physician. The homœopathic way of determining the effects of drugs by giving small doses of single, pure medicines to intelligent healthy human beings, who can observe and describe their feelings, is the only way to obtain reliable knowledge of medicines for use in healing the sick. It is safe to say that nothing of any real therapeutic value has ever been learned by experiment upon animals that could not have been learned better, more simply and more humanely by harmless experiments upon human beings; while the knowledge gained in such experiments on human beings is equally valuable for use in the treatment of sick animals.

CHAPTER XII

Examination of the Patient

We take up, in a general manner, the subject of the examination of the patient for the special purpose of making a homœopathic prescription.

At first thought it would seem as if this subject should have been presented before the general subject of symptomatology, treated in the preceding article, inasmuch as the purpose of any examination of the patient is to discover signs and symptoms. It is evident, however, that we cannot intelligently and logically take up the study of methods of examining patients for a homœopathic prescription until we have learned what symptoms are, from the homœopathic standpoint, and decided upon some adequate form of classification. We shall be more successful in our search for anything if we know what we are looking for.

The story is told of John Burroughs, the late venerable dean of American naturalists, that on one occasion he was visiting the home of an admirer, who lived in the suburbs of one of our large cities. His hostess, professing her great love of birds, bewailed their disappearance from her neighborhood. She had not seen a bird for such a long, long time. The wicked boys and the marauding cats had driven them all away! "Uncle John" looked sympathetic, but said nothing. Shortly afterward he put on his hat, tucked his note book and opera glasses in his pocket and went out for an hour's walk. On his return he invited his hostess to sit down beside him, produced his note book and showed her a list of nearly twenty different species of birds which he had observed during his hour's walk, within a half mile of her home! The difference between Mr. Burroughs and his hostess was simply that he not only knew *what* to look for, but *where* and *how* to look for it; and so he easily found what was hidden from her eyes.

So it is in examining a patient. The student who knows the

nature, constitution, forms and varieties of symptoms necessary for the homœopathic prescription will find many things in a case which another, specially trained perhaps only in pathology and general diagnosis, will entirely overlook; because pathology and diagnosis do not seek for nor take into consideration the phenomena which are most significant from the standpoint of the homœopathic prescriber. The "modalities" or "characteristic conditions," for example, which we have seen to be of the highest importance in selecting the homœopathic remedy, mean little or nothing to the pathologist or general diagnostician. The same might be said of mental and subjective symptoms. Thus we have to separate and classify the various kinds of symptoms revealed by a complete general examination, and vary our methods of examination according to the particular end in view.

The technic of an examination for the purpose of diagnosticating the disease is quite different from that of the examination for making the homœopathic prescription.

The diagnosis of disease by modern methods is based largely upon physical signs, tests and reactions, involving the use of many instruments of precision, in which the patient takes no active part, and of which he has no knowledge. The selection of the homœopathic remedy, on the other hand, is based very largely and sometimes almost entirely upon the phenomena, or deductions drawn from the phenomena, of subjective, conscious experience, perceived only by the patient and stated by him to the examiner. Nearly all of the objective phenomena possessing value from the standpoint of homœopathic therapeutics are of such a character that they require the exercise of only the physical senses and ordinary powers of observation by the patient, his friends, or the physician himself. This distinction should be kept clearly in mind. Examinations for the purpose of pathological study and for diagnosis are necessary and important in their several fields; but from the standpoint of homœopathic pharmaco-therapeutics, their importance is relative, not absolute. Aside from the physical and organic localization of disease, they furnish comparatively little that is of value to the homœopathic prescriber in his special work of selecting the symptomatically similar medicine.

Let not the pathologist, therefore, criticize the methods or findings of the prescriber, nor the diagnostician assume that his findings are sufficient for the materia-medicist; but let each regard these matters in the spirit and from the standpoint of the *physician*. For the physician, as an ideal, is greater than any medical specialist. The specialties in medicine only exist in order that, by combining them, the ideal of the perfect physician may not die and disappear from among men. However doubtful we may be of the necessity or the real value of the results, it is true that in the vast extension of so-called medical science it has become impossible for any one man to grasp and master it all. Therefore medicine has been divided into so many specialties that we might paraphrase the old proverb, "it takes nine tailors to make a man" into a new medical proverb: "It takes nine specialists to make a physician."

The general practitioner, if one dare to follow that ancient and honorable calling, must act in several capacities—as hygienist, sanitarian, pathologist, psychiatrist, diagnostician, therapeutist, and perhaps even surgeon and obstetrician; but in each of these departments he may be compelled to fill up the measure of his own technical shortcomings by recourse to the specialists. He is the wise physician who recognizes his own personal and technical limitations and judiciously uses the services of others who are specially qualified in some particular branch. And he is the wise specialist who recognizes *his* limitations—who realizes that, after all, no matter how expert he may be in his branch he is only, as it were, a part of a physician in the broad sense of the word. Modesty pays good dividends in the long run.

In this spirit we may all co-operate for the best interests of our profession and our patients, and agree with Hahnemann in the postulate of the first paragraph of the "Organon:" *"The highest and only mission of the physician is to heal the sick."* Every medical specialty is subordinate to that ideal. The work of the homœopathic prescriber, dealing specifically (as it does) with the application of medicines to disease according to a definite principle for the purpose of curing such conditions as are amenable to medicines, must ever remain one of the most important of the functions fulfilled by the physician. Although the related branches of medicine—hygiene, prophylaxis, sanitation, surgery, physical therapeutics, etc., have made great strides, the time is yet far distant when pharmaco-therapeutics will become unnecessary.

It follows that the pharmaco-therapeutist must be a specialist in the sense of becoming an expert in his department and this, let it be said, is the crying need of the profession.

With diagnostic and pathological examinations and symptoms, as such, this article has nothing to do, except to show their general relation to homœopathic prescribing. The purpose of this article is to teach the principles of "case-taking" and how to determine, from the record of an examination of a case, what symptoms are most useful as indications for the curative medicine under the homœopathic principle. Some points on the method of conducting an examination in such a manner as to discover and develop these symptoms for use in prescribing will now be presented.

In the present state of the science of pharmaco-therapeutics and with our materia medica in its present form, the most important thing to be remembered in examining a patient for a homœopathic prescription is that, with very few exceptions, the most valuable indications for the remedy are to be found:

1. In those subjective morbid sensations and phenomena which come within the sphere of the patient's own experience and are perceptible to him alone.

2. In those objective signs of disease which are perceptible to the unaided or natural senses of ourselves, the patient or others.

For the first we must, of course, depend entirely upon the statements of the patient himself. The findings of the thermometer, the stethoscope, the microscope, and the various other diagnostic instruments give us very little, as yet, that is directly available for the selection of the remedy. Their principal value is in determining the diagnosis and pathology of the case as bearing upon the prognosis and general auxiliary treatment. They also point out or more accurately define the anatomical basis of the prescription and aid us in correctly localizing symptoms.

It follows, therefore, in our special examination, that we should at once endeavor to put ourselves upon such a footing and in such personal relation to the patient as will best favor a full, frank revelation by him of all the circumstances and conditions that have led up to his illness; and an equally full, simple and frank statement of his sufferings as they seem to him. The problem is here largely psychological. It is well in some cases to briefly explain to a new patient the special purpose of a homœopathic examination and to point out how it differs from the ordinary examination, especially by including mental and subjective symptoms and certain conditions that are usually ignored.

We must first gain the patient's confidence and relieve him, as far as possible, from the sense of restraint and embarrassment. This is favored in a general way by a calm, dignified, but at the same time quiet and sympathetic manner on the part of the examiner; a demeanor confident, but not pompous; simple and direct, but not aggressive; cheerful, but not flippant; serious, but not grave or funereal. We should try to put the patient at his ease by adapting ourselves to his personality and mood.

We should not confuse the patient by a too penetrating gaze at some objective feature which may attract our attention. We may learn to observe objective phenomena accurately without seeming to do so. If a patient sees us gazing fixedly at some part of his anatomy, he is likely to become anxious and forget other matters which are of more importance to us as prescribers.

The same is true of the use of instruments and the performance of the various acts of a physical examination. A nervous patient will often be seriously disconcerted by so simple a procedure as listening to his heart action with a stethoscope—sometimes even by taking his pulse. It is best, therefore, with nervous patients, to postpone such examinations until near the close of the examination, or until he has lost his nervousness.

The patient should be encouraged to tell his story freely and relieve his mind. We want the history and symptoms of the case from the patient's standpoint first. If the physical examination is made afterward, when the patient is composed, there will be less danger of confusing or prejudicing his mind.

The first part of the examination should be conducted in an easy, semi-conversational manner. The best results, from the homœopathic standpoint, are obtained by making him forget that he is under examination. One can be painstaking and systematic without being over-formal. The mere thought of undergoing a formal examination is disconcerting to the ordinary patient. He dreads it as he dreads going to a dentist. He wants to feel, and it is best for him to feel, that he is relating his troubles to a sympathetic friend who has the resources at hand to help him. It is a good rule to keep the patient talking, but say little yourself during an examination; to let him tell his story in his own way, without interruption, except to bring him back to the subject if he digresses. We may start him in his narrative by asking when and how his trouble began, and we may instruct him to be as definite as possible in relating his history and in locating and describing his sensations *as they seem to him*. We should not laugh at him nor pedantically correct his errors.

We should not ask "leading questions," nor "put words in his mouth," but let him express his feelings and observations in his own way. Afterward, we analyze, complete, correct and interpret his statements in accordance with the principles of homœopathic symptomatology as set forth in a former article.

Notes of the patient's statements should be made while he is talking, but quietly, without ostentation.

It is well to leave a space between the symptoms as they are written so that, when the patient has finished his voluntary statement, one can glance quickly back over the page, see what has been left out and write it in. Questions are then put in such a manner as to complete each symptom as to location, sensation and modality and fill in the record.

As a matter of convenience in writing and keeping records it is well to divide the page into three vertical columns—the first for date and remedy, the second for the symptoms and the third for the modalities or conditions. This makes a page that the eye quickly takes in at a glance.

We should not hurry a patient in his narrative. We may quietly keep him to the point and prevent rambling and inconsequential statements, but that is best done, as a rule, by maintaining an attitude of business-like absorption in the medical features of the case.

It is well to keep in mind always, during the examination of a case, some working classification of symptoms—as *General, Particular* and *Common*. In examining a case we are gathering data, facts, particulars, from which we are later to determine the characteristic features of the case by the logical process of generalizing. If we are to generalize correctly we must have all the facts and be sure of them.

One thing at a time and all things in order, with an eye to the outcome. First, the analysis—facts from the patient's statements, then the nurse's, relative's or friend's statements, and then our own observations. Then comes the synthesis—the review and study of the symptoms and construction of the case, classifying symptoms as we generalize. Comparison of the symptoms of the patient with the symptoms of the materia medica in repertory work follows, and finally the selection of the indicated remedy by the exclusion process.

It is well to practice on the simple cases first, in order to become familiar with the technic. The hard cases will come soon enough and try our skill and patience to the uttermost.

The suggested classification of symptoms into general, particular and common symptoms is applicable to difficult as well as simple cases; to chronic as well as acute disease. The general plan can be modified and adapted in various ways, but the principles underlying it are always the same.

The form of the examination and the direction it takes should conform to the classification of symptoms adopted, and one may well have blanks printed to use as a guide and reminder.

Hahnemann devotes twenty-two paragraphs in the "Organon" to the subject of the examination of the patient—Paragraphs 83 to 105.

In the footnotes to these paragraphs he gives many suggestions and special directions for conducting an examination. They teach among other things, *how properly to frame our questions*—a very important matter. It is not expected that one will ask every patient all the questions which Hahnemann gives in these important footnotes, but that we shall select and apply such as bear upon the particular case in hand. They are for general guidance in the art of questioning.

There is a point in Paragraph 83 that deserves special attention for a few moments.

Hahnemann says: "This individualizing examination of a

case of disease . . . demands of the physician nothing but *freedom from prejudice* and sound senses, attention in observing and fidelity in tracing the picture of the disease."

"Without prejudice!" Said quickly it sounds simple, easy, almost trite. It is a "bitter dose" to swallow, nevertheless, when we stop to explore the depths of our own minds. In this respect it is like the old-fashioned bowl of "boneset tea" I had to swallow semi-annually in the spring and fall when I was a country boy in Wisconsin. Hot and well-sweetened it was to be sure; but bitter! Bitter was no name for it! I can still hear mother say: "Now shut your eyes, son and *swallow it quick;* then you won't taste it—much!" Sounds easy but—try it.

Who of us is without prejudice? The prejudice of a materialistic mind; of pathological theories which seem too often to be antagonistic to homœopathic principles; of doubt as to the use of the single remedy or of use of any medicine at all; the prejudice of "a constitutional aversion to work!" Many of us are "born tired." We don't like to work. Laziness, selfishness and an "easy conscience" are responsible for more homœopathic sins and shortcomings than anything else, for good homœopathic prescribing means *work!*

These are our worst enemies, and the worst enemies of homœopathy. Against these, if we are to succeed in our work, there must be a constant warfare within ourselves, until they are conquered by the establishment of correct methods and practice and a genuine interest in the work is evolved. No man who is in the grip of settled doubt or prejudice can do good work. The commercial salesman of today, for example, is not regarded as competent, nor in the proper frame of mind to gain success until he is able to *"sell himself,"* as the experts put it. That means that he must acquire and hold a thorough belief in and conviction of the usefulness, indispensability and value of the goods he has to sell. For him it means study, effort, personal self-discipline, until he develops a genuine enthusiasm for his goods, his house and his work. It means *Confidence*—in himself and in his goods.

Nowhere will prejudice show more clearly than in the homœopathic examination of a patient. If one approaches a case prejudiced in favor of some pathological theory his examination will insensibly, but inevitably, be limited by that theory. He will not get all the facts of the case, nor properly interpret those he does get; and without all the facts he cannot study or treat the case correctly.

Prejudice and doubt may be overcome by reflection, study, self-discipline and auto-suggestion; by cultivating the scientific spirit; by returning often to a consideration of and reflection upon the broad general principles underlying our art with the purpose of reforming methods, strengthening morale and correcting faulty mental attitude, or point of view; all looking toward the development of a more practical, more accurate and more comprehensive technic.

Beliefs and convictions may be strengthened and energy stimulated by reflecting upon the fact that our therapeutic method is efficient and successful because it is based upon immutable law. We may mentally recall and restate the law and its corollaries and review the facts upon which it is based, or, better yet, write a little essay on the subject; recall to mind or seek out illustrations and examples of its truth and adequacy; study the cases and cures reported in our literature by the masters; think of duty, loyalty to principle and consistency of practice; think of success, gained by right methods and without compromise. To *think success* goes a long way toward realizing success.

Our work as physicians involves the performance of a number of related functions, all of which are subordinate to the main function of healing the sick.

As specialists in therapeutic medication we examine for the symptoms upon which the choice of the remedy depends; but as physicians we also examine for the symptoms upon which the diagnosis and prognosis depends. Our aim is to make a complete examination, including all necessary pathological investigations. Having all the facts in hand we determine what features of the case are medical, what are surgical, what are psychological, what are hygienic, what are sanitary, etc. We keep all these departments distinct in our minds as bearing upon *the case as a whole*, realizing that each has its particular relations to and bearings upon all the others; and especially do we seek to realize this of the department of homœopathic therapeutics, which for us is the most important of all, because we know it is useless to attempt to base the homœopathic prescription upon anything except the symptoms which belong to its legitimate sphere. The generalizations of the diagnostician or the pathologist, be they ever so correct, cannot serve as the basis for the homœopathic prescription.

The purpose of the homœopathic examination is to bring out the symptoms of the patient in such a way as to permit of their comparison with the symptoms of the materia medica for the purpose of selecting the similar or homœopathic remedy. Every disease has its symptomatic likeness in the materia medica. The homœopathic materia medica is like a "rogues gallery" in which are hung up the portraits of all the pathological rogues in the world. When you catch a rogue compare his features with the portraits. Then make him "take his medicine!"

Like all rogue-catchers, when on duty our senses must all be on the alert, our minds clear, our logical faculties acute, our sympathies and prejudices held in abeyance. When all the facts are before us we may sympathize, correct, reassure and encourage as far as seems judicious and wise.

Artifice must sometimes be resorted to in the examination of a case, in order to get at the facts. Many obstacles have to be overcome. Among them is modesty, often on the part of the patient, *sometimes* (rarely, nowadays!) on the part of the physician if he is young and inexperienced. I often recall with amusement my feelings as I witnessed for the first time an examination of a case of phthisis pulmonalis by my old preceptor, Dr. Wells. The part of the examination which excited my risibilities was that which referred to the character of the sputum. He inquired particularly as to its color, *odor,* form and *taste!* It was the first time I had ever heard such questions and the first time that it had ever been brought home to me that such facts could have any bearing upon the selection of the remedy. I believed that I was not over modest, but such refinement of analysis rather disgusted me. After the patient had been prescribed for and dismissed, I frankly stated my difficulty to the old master. He laughed a little sympathetically at my ignorance and rallied me on my squeamishness. Then he soberly pointed out that the patient's reply that the sputum "tasted sweetish" had enabled him to differentiate between two very similar remedies and make an accurate choice. He made that the text for some sadly needed instruction in *the necessity for close analysis of all the elements of the case*—instruction which no one ever gave me during my college course.

Here, as an important part of the homœopathic examination, attention should again be directed to the use and importance of *logical analysis* in the symptomatic examination of the patient. The clinician analyzes symptoms for the same reason and by the same method that the pathologist analyzes a pathological specimen.

Many of the statements of the patient will be mere generalities. These are of no value to the prescriber until they have been analyzed into their elements. As stated, they are merely common symptoms without individuality. The patient will tell you, for example, that he has a headache. That, and all other similar generalities, must be analyzed so that the elements of locality, sensation and modality are brought out by properly framed questions. The patient may state that he has a discharge of some kind. After locating that anatomically, it should be analyzed into its elements of color, odor, consistency and quality (as bland, excoriating, causing itching, etc.). Similarly with a diarrhœa, so far as the character of the discharges are concerned; but here the act of discharge itself should be analyzed into its elements, and its character and concomitants in time and space fixed, by creating the divisions of "before stool," "during stool" and "after stool." In other words, the patient is asked to describe how he feels and what happens before, during and after the act of defecation. So in intermittent fever, for another example; the disease form is analyzed into its elements; 1. Type and periodicity (quotidian, tertian, quartan, weekly, monthly, semi-monthly, annual or semi-annual); and further as to time of day when the paroxysm appears; 2. Stages (prodrome, chill, heat, perspiration); 3. Apyrexia. In each of these divisions the phenomena are located as they appear, defining each particular symptom as accurately as possible. Thus to discover and bring out the facts of a case and give them form and individuality *as a whole,* is 'the art of the accomplished homœopathic examiner. It is an illustration of what a former article means in speaking of the "totality" as consisting of "related facts, having form, coherency and individuality," and characterizing its formation as "artistic."

Although the facts must be gathered from the patient, their form, relations and value depend almost altogether upon the examiner. The patient, unaided, will usually give only rough, disconnected statements, crude generalities, single concrete facts and a few details—a mere formless mass. The trained examiner patiently and skillfully analyzes and completes the statements, brings out details, connects the whole and constructs the case logically and scientifically, giving it a typical form, according to a preconceived idea. That is art and true art is always scientific.

As models of analysis in special diseases, and for daily practical use, procure and study Allen on Intermittent Fever; Bell on Diarrhœa and Kimball on Gonorrhœa. In general analysis and synthesis of the entire field of materia medica, Boenninghausen's "Therapeutic Pocket Book" and Kent's Repertory are classics, indispensable to every homœopathist.

Boenninghausen's "Therapeutic Pocket Book" and his book on fever (unfortunately out of print) are the original and unsuperseded models upon which all other reliable works of this class are based.

Boenninghausen, following and working with Hahnemann, is the fountain head for the analysis and classification of symptoms from which we all draw. His name, next to that of Hahnemann, is the most illustrious in the galaxy of homœopathic heroes. Methods of practice based upon and patterned after the work of such masters cannot fail to bring success to every practitioner who uses them and advance the cause of Homœopathy.

Clinical Histories.—Getting a good clinical history is one of the most important parts of case taking. By the same token it is also the one most generally neglected or badly done.

In order to deal intelligently with the present we must know something of the past. We must know not only the facts of the present, perhaps acute illness, but also what led up to it. Otherwise we will often be baffled in our attempts to cure and find our patients making slow and imperfect recoveries from seemingly simple acute diseases, or settling down into states of more or less confirmed invalidism.

This is because all genuine acute diseases are in reality acute outbreaks or exacerbations of previously latent, deep-seated, underlying, chronic diseases or inherited tendencies and predispositions to disease, which exist in practically all persons,—a special subject which is dealt with elsewhere.

In examinations then, as a rule and at the appropriate time, we first get as complete a list as possible of *the patient's previous diseases,* from childhood down to the present, in as nearly chronological order as possible, with the ages at which the attacks appeared and inquire as to their nature, symptoms, duration, severity and sequelæ.

We should inquire carefully not only as to acute eruptive, infectious, inflammatory or febrile diseases, including the so-called "children's diseases," but about the more chronic and obscure ailments, including skin diseases; organ and glandular diseases (tonsilitis, adenitis, etc.); nervous diseases (epilepsy, "convulsions," chorea, paralytic conditions, etc.); catarrhs and "discharges" from any of the mucous outlets; bone or joint diseases and rachitis; all disorders of the sexual sphere, *especially syphilis and gonorrhœa.*

In women and girls we should inquire about the menses, age at which established and regularity of the periods, note all deviations from the normal and ascertain the time and influence of marriage, childbirth, etc.

We should not forget to inquire if and when the patient *has been vaccinated* and learn what course the implanted disease took. At the same time we should inquire if any other inoculations with serums or vaccines have been performed. Many troubles may be traced back to vaccinations and inoculations, intentional or accidental.

The kind of treatment the patient has had for the diseases experienced and the principal drugs used should be learned, if possible. It may be necessary to antidote some of them.

The occupation and habits of the patient; diet, exercise, sleep, use of tea, coffee, tobacco, stimulants, narcotics, etc., should be noted.

It is important to ascertain whether the patient has met with any accidents or mechanical injuries, or has suffered any mental shock or trial, such as grief, fright, anxiety or worry, business losses or reverses, unhappy domestic experiences, disappointment in love, etc., and fix the dates and sequence. Such experiences have a powerful influence in causing or predisposing to disease besides being valuable to the prescriber as guiding symptoms.

Next it is important to ascertain the *family history*: that is, a brief history of the diseases, causes of death, predispositions and tendencies to disease and individual peculiarities not only of the patient's brothers and sisters, but of his father, mother, uncles and aunts and his grandparents, if possible.

All this is *General History* and should make up a part of the office record of every case. In some cases it will be necessary to go minutely and thoroughly into the history and phenomena of particular phases of preceding diseases in order to get the facts necessary for an intelligent homœopathic prescription.

Such an examination should be made not only for its great practical and scientific value, but for its psychological influence upon patients. Patients will be much more likely to remain permanently with the physician and his hold upon them will be much stronger if he has thorough and comprehensive histories of their cases in his files and impresses that fact upon them. It gives them confidence in his professional ability and skill.

Patients like to feel that their physician, "knows all about them;" that he is not only interested in them and their families, personally and professionally, but that he takes pains to learn and keep in touch with all their individual peculiarities. There is no surer way to build up a permanent, lucrative and substantial practice than by doing this work. It goes without saying that the fee for such a first examination must be commensurate with the time and skill employed and that it will be paid without grumbling, for every intelligent patient will see that he is getting good service and good value for his money.

Printed blanks, systematically covering the points outlined, modified according to individual judgment and need will greatly facilitate the process of good history and case taking. They should be of standard letter size, with blank sheets of the same size for expansion of individual cases and kept together, with all correspondence relating to each case, in folders, in one of the modern, indexed, vertical-filing cabinets, for constant reference. Individual records are filed alphabetically under the name of each patient. It is not well to try to keep case records on little three by four or four by five cards as some do. There should be ample space to do the subject justice. Standard letter size sheets, 8 x 10, give plenty of space, match ordinary correspondence and fit the standard vertical cabinets.

The examiner should be constantly on the alert and observing while making an oral examination. The patient may be unconscious or delirious; or an infant, unable to talk; or insane. He may be malingering or trying to deceive as to the real nature or cause of his disease. Knowledge of the natural history and phenomena of disease will aid in forming a true picture of the disease.

As a prescriber the homœopathician is always seeking that in the case which is peculiar, uncommon, characteristic, individual. That may be noticed in some casual expression of the patient as he talks, revealing his mood or state of mind, or the origin of his trouble; it may be found in the color, form, or expression of his countenance; or in his attitude, gait, or physical demeanor.

If the patient is confined to bed, the examiner will observe his position in bed, his manner of moving or turning, his respiration, the state of his skin, color or odor of perspiration, odor of exhalations from mouth or body, physical appearance of excretions, relation of the patient's sensations to atmosphere and temperature is shown in amount of covering, ventilation of room, ice bags, hot water bottle, etc.,—all these, and many other little points, noticeable by the alert examiner, perhaps without asking a question, will be valuable guides in the choice of the remedy. They should be recorded as such.

The mental state, conscious and subconscious, is revealed by the general behavior, the conversation, the expression of the countenance, the desires and aversions and the manner of sleeping, as well as by the voluntary verbal expressions. Mental symptoms are of the highest importance. Expertness in observing and analyzing these features of disease should be cultivated because right conclusions and effective treatment often depend more upon the physician's own observations and directions, than upon anything that others or even the patient are able to tell him. In the matter of mood or temper of the mind, for instance, he will be able to judge from the patient's manner of relating or expressing his sufferings and his behavior toward his attendants, whether he is sad or cheerful; calm or anxious, confident or afraid, indifferent, morose, censorious, malicious, irritable, suspicious, or jealous.

As to the intellect, he can observe for himself whether the patient is dull, stupid, unconscious, excited, delirious, distracted, confused, etc. All the foregoing points are covered by the rubrics in any good repertory and they must be covered by the remedy selected.

All these and their allied conditions are most valuable and characteristic as therapeutic indications. They should be observed and noted carefully. Every case should be approached with this thought and the mind kept active and alert while talking with the patient and his friends.

Such work as this has its pleasures, aside from its scientific relations. "The greatest study of man is man." Most of us like to "study human nature" and rather pride ourselves on our sagacity in "sizing up" the people we meet by a study of their physiognomy, manner, etc. The homœopathic prescriber will find it to his advantage to cultivate the art of psychological analysis, and may well take pride in it when he is able to do this part of his medical work systematically also.

It is taken for granted that the physical examination of a patient will be made thoroughly and systematically also and the findings added to the record. As that subject does not come within the scope of this work, no further attention will be accorded to it.

If he has succeeded in impressing upon his readers the necessity and advantages of always making thorough and systematic examinations and keeping full, written records of cases the author will feel that his purpose has been accomplished. Nothing conduces more strongly to professional honor and reputation and to success in practice. An honestly earned reputation for making careful examinations, for "taking an interest in the case," for always being thorough and painstaking, is one of the most valuable assets a physician can have, and one which may be legitimately capitalized to his financial benefit.

CHAPTER XIII

Homœopathic Posology

By posology (from the Greek, *posos,* how much) we mean the science or doctrine of *dosage*.

Small doses and homœopathy are commonly regarded as synonymous terms. If they who have such an idea of it are favorably inclined toward homœopathy, it is as likely to be because they have heard that the medicines are "pleasant to take" as for any other reason. While such an impression, taken with what it involves, is not altogether undesirable, it is to be regretted that a broader basis of judgment has not been furnished by those whose duty it is to instruct the public in the principles of homœopathy. Had this been done such a juvenile conception would not exist, and homœopathy would be more widely appreciated.

It is not to be denied that the subject of the dose in homœopathy is a very important one. The three essential elements of the system are the *principle,* the *remedy* and the *dose;* and the three are of equal importance. Posology, and the related subject of Potentiation were the subjects of so much misunderstanding, discussion and controversy in the early days of homœopathy that the profession, after being divided into two opposing camps, grew tired of the subject. It came to be regarded as a kind of "Gordian Knot," to be cut by each individual as best he could with the instrument at his disposal. Hahnemann himself at one time, almost in despair of ever being able to bring his followers to an agreement on the subject, cut the knot by proposing to treat all cases with the thirtieth potency. Following this suggestion others tacitly adopted a dosage confined to one, or a very limited range of potencies. The materialistically minded restricted themselves to the crude tinctures and triturations, or the very low dilutions, ranging from 1x to 6x. Others ranged from the third to the thirtieth potencies, while another small class of metaphysical tendency used only the very high potencies, ranging from the two hundredth to the millionth, each according to his personal predilection.

Such a state of affairs is unfortunate. Assuming that there is a difference in the action of the various doses of medicines, and that a series of potencies or preparations of the different medicines has been available for use; it follows that the entire series should be open to every practitioner, and that each man should be competent, willing and ready to use any potency or preparation of the remedy indicated in a given case, without prejudice. If he confines himself to one or two potencies, be they low, medium, or high, he is limiting his own usefulness and depriving his patient of valuable means of relief and cure.

Under homœopathic principles any potency may be required in any case. It is as unreasonable to expect to cure all cases with any two or three potencies as it is to expect to cure all cases with any two or three remedies. In either case, those who follow such a course are governed more by the love of ease and their prejudices than they are by their desire for efficiency.

The selection of the dose is as much an integral part of the process of making a homœopathic prescription as the selection of the remedy, and often quite as important. A well selected remedy may fail utterly, or even do injury, because of wrong dosage. Dose as well as remedy must be adjusted to the patient's need.

The homœopathic doctrine of dosage, like the law of cure, was based upon the discovery of the *opposite action of large and small doses of medicine*. It is another application in medicine of the Law of Mutual Action—the third Newtonian law of motion—"Action and Reaction are Equal and Opposite." Every one at all acquainted with the action of drugs knows, for example, that Ipecac in large doses causes nausea and vomiting and in small doses, under certain conditions, will cure the same; that Opium in large doses will cause a deep sleep or narcosis, and in small doses, under certain conditions, will cure the same.

Closely allied to this is the so-called primary and secondary action of drugs, in which we see many drugs, in the first or primary stage of their action producing one group of symptoms, and in the second stage a directly opposite set of phenomena; as when the deep sleep of the primary action of Opium is followed by a much longer lasting wakefulness; or where the diarrhœa induced by a cathartic is followed by a longer lasting constipation. This applies, of course, only to drugs given in tangible form and considerable quantities, in what are called "physiological doses."

Although the physiological antagonism between large and small doses is an illustration of the homœopathic law of posology, the use of drugs in "physiological doses" has nothing to do with their homœopathic use, because *homœopathic remedies are never used in "physiological doses."* This statement is true, even in those cases where the low reacting power of the patient sometimes requires *material doses* of the homœopathic remedy. It would be more accurate to say that homœopathic medicines are never used for their *"physiological effect."*

It is necessary to a clear understanding of the subject that a distinction be made between three terms, physiological, therapeutic, and pathogenetic, used by the two schools of medicine to express the nature of the action of the drugs. There is a demoralizing tendency even in the homœopathic school to use these terms without discrimination.

The word "physiological" as currently used in medicine in relation to drug action and dosage is misleading and inaccurate. The word has a reassuring sound, pleasantly suggestive of something normal and healthy. Its use tends to obscure, or keep in the background, the fact that the kind of drug action so designated is essentially a *toxic* action and therefore really painful and injurious.

The "physiological action" of a drug is not its therapeutic or curative action. It is exactly the opposite of a curative action, and is never employed in homœopathic practice for therapeutic purposes. The use of the word "physiological" in connection with drug action and drug dosage tends to mislead the unwary and justify the use of measures which would otherwise be regarded as illegitimate. In one word, is it a euphemism. Inasmuch as the action of the "physiological" dose and the purpose for which it is given is avowedly to *produce drug symptoms,* in a direct and positive manner, that fact should be clearly expressed in the name, in order that there may be no misunderstanding.

The homœopathic school has recognized the wisdom and

justice of taking this position, and has complied with the requirements of scientific accuracy in nomenclature by the adoption and use of the word "pathogenetic" (Gr., *pathos,* suffering, and *genesis,* origin, "producing suffering") as properly describing the character of such drug action. The "suffering" of the organism produced by the drug is expressed in symptoms, which are the language of disease. In homœopathic parlance, therefore, these are termed "pathogenetic symptoms," a term which is preferable because it is accurate and truthful.

Therapeutic means curative, healing, alleviating. A pathogenetic action is never curative. The action of a drug may be pathogenetic (toxic), or therapeutic (curative), depending upon the size and strength of the dose, the susceptibility of the patient and the principle upon which it is given.

In the homœopathic treatment of disease a drug is never given for its pathogenetic action. Pathogenetic doses may be given, however, for experimental purposes to a healthy person, in making what are called provings. In treating disease homœopathically the object is not to *produce symptoms* but to *remove them.* By means of the similar remedy in the minimum dose it is possible to do this in a direct manner without producing symptoms. It is not necessary to resort to the indirect, antipathic or allopathic method of producing drug symptoms in one part to remove a disease of the same, or any other part, and therefore it is not necessary to use "physiological" or pathogenetic doses. The homœopathic cure is obtained without suffering, without the production of any drug symptoms, in a positive and direct manner, by the action of sub-physiological or sub-pathogenetic doses; in other words, by the *minimum dose,* which is a dose so small that it is not capable of producing symptoms when used therapeutically. Homœopathy requires that the therapeutic dose must be capable only of producing a slight temporary aggravation or intensification of *already existing symptoms,* never of producing new symptoms. Only the similar remedy, in the smallest possible dose, is capable of bringing about this highly desirable result. By this means the patient's strength and vitality are conserved, his suffering quickly reduced to the lowest possible degree and a true cure brought about, if the case has not passed beyond the curative stage. It is not to be understood that infinitesimal doses are not capable of producing symptoms in healthy susceptible persons; for that is not true. Infinitesimal doses will produce symptoms in certain highly sensitive persons, and many of our most valuable provings have been made with more or less highly potentiated medicines. Indeed, no remedy can be regarded as having been thoroughly proven until it has been proven in the potencies as well as in crude form.

In ordinary usage a physiological dose means a dose of a drug, empirically selected, of sufficient quantity and strength to produce a definite, predetermined effect or group of symptoms. Practically it amounts to the *maximum dose* consistent with safety. A physiological dose of Atropine or Belladonna, for example, is one sufficient to produce dilatation of the pupils, dryness of the mucous membranes and flushing or turgescence of the skin. The action of the drug is carried to this point irrespective of any accessory symptoms that may be produced, or as to whether it is curative or otherwise. No other kind of action is looked for or expected and, as a rule, it is not recognized if it occurs. The intent is to produce a direct definite drug effect. That other effects not desired nor needed are produced incidentally, does not matter. They are left to take care of themselves, and it is not considered that they complicate or prejudice the case if they occur.

In attempting to predetermine arbitrarily the size and strength of the physiological dose, allowance is made only for difference in the age of the patients, who are roughly divided into two classes, infants and adults. If a patient is unable to take the established or usual doses without serious results, it is considered to be a case of idiosyncrasy or hypersensitiveness and some other drug is substituted.

Unlike the homœopathic physician, the allopathic practitioner is not trained to observe the finer, more delicate action of drugs upon the living organism and he does not, therefore, recognize the symptoms expressing such actions when they occur. From this point of view such symptoms, so long as they are not serious, are of no importance and have no use.

In considering the reasons why the dose of the medicine chosen homœopathically is necessarily smaller than the physiological dose of antipathic or allopathic prescription, we meet first the fact of *organic resistance*.

Every living organism is endowed with an inherent, automatic power of reaction to stimuli. By means of this power the organism offers resistance to everything which tends to injure or destroy its integrity or disturb its normal functioning. Resistance is manifested by suffering, pain, fever, inflammation, changed secretions and excretions, etc.

This power is displayed when drugs are administered because drugs are inimical to health, in proportion to their power and the size of the dose. In order for a dissimilar drug to produce its so-called physiological effect, therefore, the dose must be large enough to overcome first, this bodily resistance; and second, to produce its characteristic symptoms.

When the similar or homœopathic drug is administered in disease, little or no resistance is encountered, because the sphere of its action has already been invaded and its resistance overcome by the similarly acting disease producing agent. The affected organs or tissues are open to attacks from without. Susceptibility to the similar drug is therefore greatly increased.

The homœopathic drug acts upon the identical tracts involved in the disease process, in a manner similar to the action of the disease producing cause itself. In order that the suffering of the affected organs may not be increased and the patient injured, a much smaller dose must be given.

The homœopathic dose, therefore, is always a sub-physiological or sub-pathogenetic dose; that is, a dose so small as not to produce pathogenetic symptoms; for we desire, not to produce more symptoms, but only to remove and obliterate symptoms already existing. It must also be given in a dose so small as not to produce a severe aggravation of the already existing symptoms.

Another reason for the small dose lies in the fact that disease renders the affected parts abnormally sensitive, as we see in an inflamed eye, which is painfully sensitive to a degree of light to which it reacts normally in health.

A third reason is that the homœopathic drug is always given singly, so that its action is complete and unmodified by other drugs.

Homœopathists do not say, vaguely, that medicines in infinitesimal doses cure disease unconditionally. The proposition is that medicines act curatively in infinitesimal quantities, *when given in cases to which they are homœopathic*. And they still further qualify this statement by laying down three necessary requirements for such action:—

1. The development of special virtues in medicine by a peculiar process of preparation, or potentiation.
2. The increased susceptibility to medicinal impression produced by disease.
3. The selection of the symptomatically similar remedy.

They affirm and stand ready to demonstrate that an infinitesimal dose of medicine *has power* and that it acts as *a force;* but in order that the force should be medicinal, or curative, a condition of application is necessary; namely, that it be applied in accordance with the homœopathic law.

Force, to be effective, must be supplied not only in proper amount, but in the proper direction and at the proper time.

The proper amount of a drug to be administered in a given case can never be settled by *a priori* reasoning, but only by experience; and thus it has been settled. Those who hesitate to try the infinitesimal doses of homœopathy on the ground of improbability, should be reminded that an infinitesimal quantity *is a quantity*. It cannot be thought of as *nothing*. Hear Hahnemann's reply to those who railed at the infinitesimal dose as "Nothing," and "Absurd."

"How so? The smallest possible portion of a substance, is it not an integral part of the whole? Were it to be divided and redivided even to the limits of infinity, would there not still remain *something*,—something *substantial*,—a part of the whole, let it be ever so minute? What man in his senses would deny it?

And if this be in reality an integral part of the divided substance, which no man in his senses can doubt, why should this minute portion, as it is certainly *something*, be *inactive*, while the whole acted with so much violence?"

Hahnemann's final views and practice in regard to the dose were arrived at gradually, through long years of careful experiment and observation; at first, even for some time after the promulgation of the law of similars and the method of practice based upon it, he used medicines in material doses and in the usual form. His discovery of the principle of potentiation came about gradually as he experimented in the reduction of his doses, in order, to arrive at a point where severe aggravations would not occur. Gradually, by experience, he learned that the latent powers of drugs were released or developed by trituration, dilution and succussion. Thus he arrived at his final conclusion that *the proper dose is always the least possible dose which will effect a cure.*

Having now a general view of the principles underlying the question of the dose, and a general standard by which to test results, it is desirable to try to formulate some rules, based upon experience, to govern us in the selection of the proper dose for a particular case.

The question seems more complex now than it was in Hahnemann's day, but really it is not so. The same principle applies now as then. For the greater part of his life Hahnemann had only what we now call the lower potencies; namely from the first to the thirtieth; although in his later years he was enabled to procure and use some of the higher potencies. Boenninghausen wrote that Hahnemann had repeatedly stated to him that he generally used the sixtieth dilution, and that he often used much higher ones with great satisfaction. Boenninghausen also states that Hahnemann, in correspondence with him, was much interested in the experiments of Boenninghausen and Gross with the high potencies and heartily approved of the same. It was repeatedly stated that Hahnemann would deal with this subject in the forthcoming sixth edition of the Organon, a work which unfortunately never saw the light until 1922.

Since Hahnemann's day the potency makers have been busy and we now have potencies ranging up to the millionth centesimal, and ever higher. Men with the confidence, courage and zeal to experiment with these altitudinous preparations and publish their results have not been lacking. Physicians of unquestioned honesty, ability and experience have testified that they obtained curative results from the use even of the very highest potencies. It is not just for us to question this testimony until we have put the matter to the test. In the light of experience and of recent revelations in other departments of science of the power of the infinitesimal, there is nothing inherently improbable about it, and it is unquestionably to our advantage to have as large an armamentarium as possible.

The great bulk of the work of the profession, however, is done with the lower and medium potencies and these, if accurately prescribed and wisely managed, will give satisfactory results in the great majority of cases. The third, sixth, twelfth and thirtieth potencies with a set of the two hundredths to "top off with" gives a general working range. When the young practitioner can afford to add to these a set of BOERICKE & TAFEL'S hand made five hundredths and one thousandths, he will be well equipped indeed. The rest is "velvet;" but if anybody should offer him a set of Fincke's, Swan's or Skinner's fifty thousandths and one hundred thousandths, he should not let his modesty nor his prejudices prevent him from accepting and trying them. Hundreds of practitioners, including the writer, have used them with great satisfaction.

Choosing the Potency.—Now is there any teaching which will help us to choose the best potency for a given case? There is little teaching but many opinions. Practitioners who publicly boast of their liberality on this subject, will too often be found, on more intimate acquaintance, to practice an obstinate exclusivism in the use of some particular potency, generally a very low or a very high one; and to harshly criticize those who differ with them. This is unfortunate, because such practitioners undoubtedly deprive themselves and their patients of many agents of cure which are easily within their reach.

The series of potencies has been compared to the gamut in music, "A skillful artist may indeed construct a harmony with the various vibrations of the same chord; but what a more beautiful and perfect harmony might he construct by a proper combination of all the sounds that can be elicited from his instrument." (Guernsey.)

In general it may be stated that any curable diseases may be cured by any potency, when the indicated remedy is administered; but that the cure may be much accelerated by selecting the potency or dose appropriate to the individual case.

Five considerations influence us in the choice of the dose:
1. The susceptibility of the patient.
2. The seat of the disease.
3. The nature and intensity of the disease.
4. The stage and duration of the disease.
5. The previous treatment of the disease.

Susceptibility of the Patient.—This is generally and rightly regarded as the most important guide in the selection of the dose. It is important to have some means of gauging, at least approximately, the susceptibility of a patient.

Susceptibility to medicinal action is only a part or phase of the general susceptibility of the organism to all stimuli. By analogy, as well as by experience, we are led to a consideration of the main factors which modify and express susceptibility in general.

Susceptibility varies in different individuals according to age, temperament, constitution, habits, character of diseases and environment.

The susceptibility of an individual to a remedy at different times also varies. Idiosyncrasy may exist as a modifying factor. Homœopathicity must always be considered.

The more similar the remedy, the more clearly and positively the symptoms of the patient take on the peculiar and characteristic form of the remedy, the greater the susceptibility to that remedy, and the higher the potency required.

The "Indefatigable Jahr" has very lucidly and beautifully illustrated this point. He remarks an essential difference between the action of the low and high potencies, which consists, not in their strength or weakness, but in the *development of the peculiarities of the remedy, as we rise in the scale of potencies.* This is based on the well known fact that provings of the tincture and lowest potencies of a drug, as a rule, produce only the more common and general symptoms of the drug, not very sharply differentiated from other drugs of its class. It is in the provings of the medium and higher potencies that the special and peculiar character of the drug is revealed by its finer and most characteristic symptoms. Jahr illustrates this by a geometrical figure, consisting of a number of concentric circles, with radii drawn to represent remedies in different stages of potentiation.

In the first to the third potency, as shown in the innermost circle where the radii lie close together, similar or related remedies like Ars., Rhus, Bry., and Sulph., have a great many symptoms in common; but the higher they progress in the scale of potentiation the more the radii recede from each other, so that each appears more and more distinctly in its peculiar and characteristic features.

All narcotics, like Bell., Stram., or Opium, for example, in crude and massive doses act in a manner equally stupefying, causing death by apoplexy or paralysis; all drastics produce vomiting and purging, etc. It is only in small or potentiated doses that their most characteristic differences of action become apparent.

"By continual diluting and succussing," says Jahr, "remedies get neither stronger nor weaker, but their individual peculiarities become more and more developed;" in other words, *their sphere of action is enlarged,* as represented by the concentric circles.

The practical bearing of this on the selection of the potency or dose, according to Jahr, is as follows:—In a given case, where the symptoms are not clearly developed and there is an absence or scarcity of characteristic features; or where two or three remedies seem about equally indicated, susceptibility and reaction may be regarded as low. We give, therefore, the remedy which seems most similar, in a low (third to twelfth) potency. But when the symptoms of a case clearly indicate one remedy, whose characteristic symptoms correspond closely to the characteristic symptoms of the case, we give the high potencies—thirtieth, two hundredth, thousandth, or higher, according to the prescriber's degree of confidence and the contents of his medicine case.

We may slightly modify Jahr's advice by suggesting; the clearer and more positively *the finer, more peculiar and more characteristic symptoms of the remedy appear* in a case, the higher the degree of susceptibility and the higher the potency.

This rule covers more points of the requirements to be stated later than appears at first glance. The class of cases (to be described later) which require low potencies for their cure, do not as a rule present the finest and most characteristic shadings of symptoms which characterize the cases requiring high potencies; so that we may pretty safely judge the degree of susceptibility of the patient by the character and completeness of the symptoms.

Allowance should be made, however, for the varying ability of examiners. One man, keen of perception, accurate, painstaking, conscientious and well trained, will see many things in a case which another not so endowed will fail to see.

Susceptibility is Modified by Age.—Generally speaking, susceptibility is greatest in children and young, vigorous persons, and diminishes with age. Children are particularly sensitive during development, and the most sensitive organs are those which are being developed. Therefore the medicines which have a peculiar affinity for those organs should be given in the medium or higher potencies.

Susceptibilty is Modified by Constitution and Temperament.—The higher potencies are best adapted to sensitive persons of the nervous, sanguine or choleric temperament; to intelligent, intellectual persons, quick to act and react; to zealous and impulsive persons.

Lower potencies and larger and more frequent doses correspond better to torpid and phlegmatic individuals, dull of comprehension and slow to act; to coarse fibered, sluggish individuals of gross habits; to those who possess great muscular power but who require a powerful stimulus to excite them. Such persons can take with seeming impunity large amounts of stimulants like whiskey, and show little effect from it. When ill they often require low potencies or even, sometimes, material doses.

Susceptibility is Modified by Habit and Environment.—It is increased by intellectual occupation, by excitement of the imagination and emotions, by sedentary occupations, by long sleep, by an effeminate life. Such persons require high potencies.

Susceptibility is Modified by Pathological Conditions.—In certain terminal conditions the power of the organism to react, even to the indicated homœopathic remedy, may become so low that only material doses can arouse it. A common example of this is seen in certain terminal conditions of valvular heart disease, where Digitalis is the indicated remedy, but no effect is produced by any potency. The patient will respond, however, to tangible doses of the pure tincture or a fresh infusion of Digitalis and sometimes make a good recovery from a condition that seems hopeless. Although such doses, judged only by their amount, might be regarded as "physiological" or pathogenetic doses, the nature of the reaction in such cases is clearly not pathogenetic but dynamic and curative, as many have witnessed. The form of the reaction complies perfectly with the requirements of cure as to order and direction of the disappearance of the symptoms and nature of the result.

Quantity alone does not constitute a pathogenetic dose. Quality, proportionality and the susceptibility of the patient are also factors. What would be a large, injurious or perhaps dangerous dose for a highly susceptible patient, would have no effect whatever upon one whose power to react was very low by reason of the existence of gross pathological lesions, or of long existant, exhausting chronic disease and much previous treatment. *It is solely a question of approximating the quality and quantity of the dose to the grade or plane of the disease, according to the law of similars.* If the grade of the disease is low, and the power of reaction low, the remedy must be given low. Thus we find, in such cases, that the symptoms of the patient are usually of a low order; common, pathological symptoms; organ symptoms; gross terminal symptoms; symptoms that correspond to the effects of crude drugs in massive toxic doses. The finer shadings of symptoms belonging to acute conditions, in vigorous sensitive patients, do not appear. Potentiated medicines will not act. The case has passed beyond that stage, and the finer symptoms with it. Yet the symptoms remain and the almost hopeless conditions they represent, are still within the scope of the homœopathic law; and they sometimes yield to its power, when the related law of posology is rightly understood and applied.

So-called "pathological symptoms," when they exist alone, are as significant and characteristic in their way and may be as clearly indicative of a remedy, homœopathically, as the earlier, finer grades of symptoms. Whether they are as useful to the homœopathic prescriber or not *depends upon the existence of similar symptoms in the Materia Medica.* We can only prescribe for symptoms which have a counterpart in the Materia Medica. From the records of poisonings, over-dosing, and some extreme provings, as well as from clinical experience, we have knowledge of some drugs whose symptoms thus derived, correspond very closely to the class of pathological symptoms under discussion. In the list of such drugs we may find one which fits our case. If that is not possible a study of the *early symptoms* from the history of the case, if they can be elicited, may lead directly or by analogy, to the remedy needed. When a case has reached a stage where none but gross pathological or organ symptoms are present, it is usually incurable; but it is not necessarily beyond help by medicines homœopathically selected, even if no results follow the use of the ordinary small doses or potentiated medicines.

In terminal conditions, therefore, when the patient does not react to well selected remedies, nor to intercurrent reaction remedies, given in potentiated form and small doses, resort to the crude drug and increase the dose to the point of reaction.

When reasonably sure of the remedy give the tincture, or a low trituration, first in moderate, then in increasing doses until the dosage is found to which the patient will react, even if it be the "maximum dose" as set down in the books. The "maximum dose" may be the "minimum dose" necessary to bring about reaction sometimes. It takes more power to drive an automobile up a hill than it does on the level; and if the hill is very steep the driver may have to go backward on the road a ways and take "a running start," in order to gain momentum enough to carry him up. When he gets to the top of the hill he can shut off power and "coast" down the other side. That is what the homœopathic prescriber has to do sometimes, in the kind of cases under discussion.

This does not in the least degree invalidate nor violate the principle of the minimum dose in such cases. The principle of *similia* as applied in the selection of both remedy and dose is eternally and universally true. It is as true in terminal conditions in chronic diseases marked by gross pathological lesions and symptoms as it is in any other kind of cases. The homœopathic physician fails and falls short of his duty if, at such a crisis, he throws up his hands and lets his patient die or pass into other hands; or if he weakly yields, abandons the principle of *similia* and resorts to the routine measures of allopathic practice, based upon theoretical assumptions. Occasionally an allopathic physician is called in who gives so-called physiological doses of some common drug and restores the patient. He merely does what the homœopathic physician should have the discernment and common sense to do;—namely, give the drug that is *really homœopathic to the case*, but give it in the stronger doses required at that stage of the case to excite the curative reaction. He does what the homœopathic physician is perhaps too timid, too ignorant or too prejudiced to do. Result: the allopath gets the honor, the family and the emolument; the homœopath "gets the laugh;" and homœopathy "gets a black eye." The occasional successes of allopathic physicians in such cases are nearly always accomplished with drugs which are essentially, although crudely, homœopathic. The homœopath who habitually uses high potencies is apt to forget or overlook the fact that a terminal case may reach a point where the symptoms call for material doses because the susceptibility is so low that it will react to no other, but will react to them.

Such a case occurred in the practice of the writer. It was a case of valvular heart disease of many years' standing, which had reached the stage of fibrillation. In a previous crisis it had responded to potentiated medicines. In this instance, however, potentiated medicines, selected with the greatest care, had no effect. An effort was made to arouse the dormant reactivity with intercurrent remedies, also in high potency. Laurocerasus, Carbo vegetabilis, Tuberculinum and Medorrhinum were given, as recommended by homœopathic authorities.

All efforts failed and the case rapidly progressed toward dissolution. Tachycardia, arrhythmia, œdema, ascites, hydrothorax, passive congestion of the brain and liver, delirium, suppression of urine and coma foretold the rapid approach of the end. For a period of over three weeks the symptoms had positively and unmistakably demanded Digitalis; but doses ranging from forty thousandth down to drop doses of the tincture produced no favorable change.

At this point, by advice of an eminent allopathic specialist who was called in at the request of the family, full doses of a special preparation of Digitalis and a salt-free, liquid diet were given. Within thirty-six hours the patient was passing over one hundred ounces of urine in twenty-four hours, brain, lungs and liver rapidly cleared up and the case which had appeared absolutely hopeless progressed steadily to a good recovery.

The action of the Digitalis was clearly curative. No pathogenetic symptoms of any kind appeared, for the copious urine was distinctly a curative symptom. Only six doses of the drug were given, at intervals of twelve hours, and it was discontinued as soon as its full therapeutic action was established.

About one month later, it was necessary to repeat the medication in smaller doses a few times for a slight return of some of the symptoms, due to over exertion.

This patient was not cured in the sense that his structurally damaged heart valves were restored, for that is an impossibility. But the action of the indicated drug was curative in its nature, as far as it was possible to go, his life was saved and prolonged, and he was restored to a measure of comfort and usefulness, when otherwise he would have died.

Digitalis in material doses was homœopathic to his condition, symptomatically and pathologically and no other drug could take its place at that stage of the disease. No other medicine of any kind was given.

In contrast to this case, and in further illustration of the necessity for being prepared to use the entire scale of potencies, the following case from the practice of the writer is presented.

The patient was a girl eighteen years of age, in the late stages of incurable heart disease. She had been under allopathic treatment for over a year, steadily growing worse. When first seen by the writer she was confined to a chair, unable to lie down or remain in bed. General œdema, ascites and hydrothorax existed. Urine was almost entirely suppressed, only about four ounces being passed in twenty-four hours. Tachycardia and dyspnœa were most distressing and death seemed imminent. The history and anamnesis of her case revealed unmistakable Calcarea symptoms. She was given a single dose of Calcarea carb., C.M., Fincke. The reaction and response to the remedy was surprising. Within forty-eight hours urine began to be secreted copiously. For several days she passed from one hundred and twenty to one hundred and fifty ounces per day. Dropsy rapidly disappeared and she was soon able to lie down and sleep comfortably. In about four weeks she was able to go out for a ride in a carriage, and not long after was out walking. She lived thirteen months in comparative comfort and happiness and then died quite suddenly of heart failure, after a slight over exertion.

These two cases represent the extremes of therapeutic resources open to the homœopathic practitioner.

Susceptibility is Modified by Habit and Environment.— People who are accustomed to long and severe labor out-of-doors, who sleep little and whose food is coarse, are less susceptible.

Persons exposed to the continual influence of drugs, such as tobacco workers and dealers; distillers and brewers and all connected with the liquor and tobacco trade; druggists, perfumers, chemical workers, etc., often possess little susceptibility to medicines and usually require low potencies in the illnesses, except where their illness is directly caused by some particular drug influence, when a high potency of the same or a similar drug may prove to be the best antidote.

Idiots, imbeciles and the deaf and dumb have a low degree of susceptibility, as a rule.

"There is no rule without its exceptions" and this is especially true in this matter of the homœopathic doses. Contrary to what one would expect, persons who have taken many crude drugs of allopathic, homœopathic or "bargain-counter" prescription often require high potencies for their cure. Their susceptibility to crude drugs and low potencies has been exhausted and even massive doses seem to have no effect; as where cathartics or anodynes have been used until there is no reaction to them. Such cases will often respond at once to high potencies of the indicated remedy; in fact they often require the high potency as an antidote. The high potency is effective because it acts on virgin soil, invades new territory, as it were.

When the old "Chronics" begin to come in to see the New Doctor—"old rounders" upon whom the contents of the drug shops and the medicine cases of his tincture and low potency competitors have been exhausted in vain—"an' he be wise" he will get out his little high potency case and prescribe from that. The results will surprise them, if it does not surprise him. It should not surprise him because he has been told before hand.

The seat, character, and intensity of the disease has some bearing upon the question of the dose. Certain malignant and rapidly fatal diseases, like cholera, may require material doses or low potencies of the indicated drug. Hahnemann's famous prescription of Camphor in drop doses of the strong tincture, given every five or ten minutes, with which so many thousands of lives have been saved, is an illustration. Later, after reaction has been established and other remedies, corresponding to the symptoms of later stages of the disease come into view, the higher potencies are required.

Generally speaking, *diseases characterized by diminished vital action require the lower potencies; while diseases characterized by increased vital action respond better to high potencies;* but this again is modified by the temperament and constitution of the patient. Uncomplicated, typical syphilis, in its primary stage, the chancre still being existent, may be cured speedily by Mercury in medium or high potencies, if the patient is of the nervous or sanguine temperament, and especially if he has not already received treatment. If he is of the sluggish type, however, Mercury in the second or third trituration will probably be required. If the patient presents himself later, having already received the conventional large doses of mercury and potash until the characteristic dynamic and pathogenetic symptoms of those drugs have been produced, low potencies will be of no avail. Either susceptibility has been exhausted, or a drug idiosyncrasy has been developed. The drugs must be antidoted and the further treatment carried on by higher potencies. These remarks apply not only to mercury and syphilis but to practically all other diseases and drugs. It is not to be inferred that mercury is the only remedy for syphilis; for in syphilis, as in all other diseases, we must individualize both case and remedy, if we expect to cure our patients.

What has been said of the use of higher potencies in cholera, after reaction has been established by camphor tincture, is applicable in many other diseases of malignant character and rapid progress. In the beginning, when torpor or collapse indicate the dangerously low vitality and deficient reaction, a few doses of a low potency may be required until reaction comes about, after which the potency should be changed to a higher one if it is necessary to repeat the remedy. The question is entirely one of susceptibility. The higher the susceptibility, the higher the potency. We must learn how to judge the degree of susceptibility if we would be successful as homœopathic prescribers; and this applies not only to the normal susceptibility of the patient as evidenced by his constitution, temperament, etc., but to the varying degrees of his susceptibility as modified by the character and stages of his disease and by previous treatment. At one stage he may need a low potency, as already pointed out, and at another a high potency. The man who confines himself to the use of a single potency, or two or three potencies, be they low or high, is not availing himself of all the measures of his art and will frequently fail to cure.

Attempts have been made to lay down rules governing the dose based upon a pathological classification of diseases; as, for example, that the lower preparations should be used in chronic disease with tendency to disorganization of tissues and in acute diseases; or that the high potencies should be used in purely functional and nervous affections; but these classifications are not reliable. They only serve to confuse the mind of the student and distract his attention from the main point, *which is to determine the degree of susceptibility of the particular patient at a given time.*

Thus the whole matter of the dose, like the selection of the remedy, resolves itself into *a problem of individualization,* which, as a principle, governs all the practical operations of homœopathy. Looking at this subject broadly and having the highest degree of success in view, it is seen that it is as necessary to individualize the dose as it is the remedy, and that the whole scale of potencies must be open to the prescriber.

Occasionally a case will be met which is not at all susceptible to the indicated remedy. In such cases the temporary insensibility to medicine may be traced to the previous abuse of medicine, or to an exciting regimen. If time and the exigencies of the case permit, it is sometimes best to cease all medication for a few days and carefully regulate the diet and regimen. Then medication may be resumed, using, according to the temperament and constitution of the patient, either a low or a medium potency.

Hahnemann has recommended in such cases, the administration of Opium, in one of the lowest potencies, every eight or twelve hours until some signs of reaction are perceptible. By this means, he says, the susceptibility is increased and new symptoms of the disease are brought to light. Carbo veg., Laurocerasus, Sulphur and Thuja are other remedies suited to such conditions. They sometimes serve to arouse the organism to reaction so that indicated remedies will act.

Remedies used in this way are known as "Intercurrents." The nosodes, Psorinum, Syphilinum, Medorrhinum, Tuberculinum, are also to be remembered in this condition, in cases where the latent diseases represented by these medicines are present, as shown by the existent symptoms or by the history and previous symptoms of the case. A single dose of the appropriate nosode in a moderately high potency, will sometimes clear up a case by bringing symptoms into view which will make it possible to select the remedy required to carry on the case successfully. Such use of remedies must be based upon a careful examination and study of the history of the case and not merely upon empirical assumptions. Here, as elsewhere, individualization and the law of *similia* must guide.

Repetition of Doses.—It remains to speak of one more important matter connected with the general subject of Homœopathic Posology—the repetition of the dose. The management of the remedy in regard to potency and dosage is almost as important as the selection of the remedy itself. The selection of the remedy can hardly be said to be finished until the potency and dosage have been decided upon. These three factors, remedy, potency and dosage, are necessarily involved in the operation of prescribing. Not one of them is a matter of indifference and not one of them can be disregarded.

The first question which confronts us is whether to give one dose or repeated doses. The second question is, if we give one dose when shall we repeat it? Third, if we give repeated doses, how often shall we repeat the doses and when shall we stop dosing?

Many expert prescribers begin the treatment of practically all cases by giving a single dose of the indicated remedy and awaiting reaction. This is an almost ideal method—for expert prescribers. Of course we all expect to become expert prescribers and will therefore accept that as our ideal!

Hahnemann's usual teaching, the outcome of his long and rich experience, was to give a single dose and await its full action. The wisdom of this teaching has been amply confirmed since his day by many of his followers. The duration of action of a remedy *which acts* (and no other counts) varies, of course, with the nature and rate of progress of the disease. In a disease of such violence and rapid tendency toward death as cholera, for example, the action of the indicated remedy might be exhausted in five or ten minutes and another dose be required at the end of that time. In a slowly progressing chronic disease, like tuberculosis, the action of a dose of a curative remedy might continue for two or three months. Between these two extremes are all degrees of variation.

The only rule which can be laid down with safety is to *repeat the dose only when improvement ceases*. To allow a dose, or a remedy, to act as long as the improvement produced by it is sustained, is good practice; but to attempt to fix arbitrary limits to the action of medicine, as some have done, is contrary to experience.

Young practitioners and many old ones too, for that matter, give too many doses, repeat too frequently, change remedies too often. They give no time for reaction. They get doubtful, or hurried, or careless and presently they get "rattled" if the case is serious. Then it is "all up with them," until or unless they come to their senses and correct their mistakes. Sometimes such mistakes cannot be corrected and a patient pays the penalty with his life. It pays to be careful and "go slow" in the beginning; then there will not be so many mistakes to correct. We should examine our case carefully and systematically, select our first remedy and potency with care, give our first dose, if the single dose is decided upon and then watch results. If the remedy and dose are right *there will be results*. We need have no doubt on that score. The indicated remedy and potency, even in a single dose cannot be given without some result and the result must be good. Generally speaking, it may be taken for granted that if there is no perceptible result after a reasonable time, depending upon the nature of the case, either the remedy or the potency was wrong.

One of the most difficult things is to *learn to wait*. Three things are necessary; wisdom, courage and patience. "Strong doses" and frequent repetition will not avail if the remedy is not right.

In Par. 245 Hahnemann gives this general rule: *"Perceptible and continued progress of improvement in an acute or chronic disease, is a condition which, as long as it lasts, invariably counterindicates the repetition of any medicine whatever,* because the beneficial effect which the medicine continues to exert is rapidly approaching its perfection. Under these circumstances every new dose of medicine would disturb the process of recovery."

In the long note to Par. 246, however, which should be carefully studied, Hahnemann qualifies this statement and indicates the circumstances under which it is advisable to repeat the doses of the same remedy, using the action of Sulphur in chronic diseases as an illustration.

In Pars. 247-8, Hahnemann says: "These periods" (marked by the repetition of doses) *"are always to be determined by the more or less acute course of the disease and by the nature of the remedy employed.* The dose of the same medicine is to be repeated several times, if necessary, but only until recovery ensues, or until the remedy ceases to produce improvement; at that period the remainder of the disease, having suffered a change in its group of symptoms, requires another homœopathic medicine." Study also Pars. 249-252.

The single dose of the indicated remedy, repeated whenever improvement ceases, as long as new or changed symptoms do not indicate a change of remedy, is adapted to all cases, but especially to chronic cases and to such acute cases as can be seen frequently and watched closely. The nature and progress of the disease will determine, under this rule, how often the dose is to be repeated. Cases may present themselves, however, which cannot be watched as closely as we would like. We may not be able to visit the patient frequently, nor remain with him long enough to observe the full period of remedial action. In such cases it is permissible and indeed necessary, to order a repetition of doses at stated intervals of one, two, or three hours, until improvement is felt or seen, or perhaps until our next visit. In such cases it is well to direct that the medicine be stopped as soon as the patient is better, giving some simple instruction to the nurse as to what constitutes a reliable sign of improvement, according to the nature of the case.

If a patient is so gravely ill as to require doses at intervals of less than one hour it is the physician's duty to remain with the patient and judge of his condition and progress for himself, *unless he is absolutely sure of the remedy,* or is in telephonic communication with the case.

Effect of the Remedy.—The next point to be considered under the general subject of Homœopathic Posology is: *The Effect of the Remedy.*

After we have selected what we believe to be the indicated remedy and administered it in proper potency and dosage, it is our duty to observe the patient carefully in order that we may correctly note and intelligently interpret the changes that occur; for upon these changes in the patient's condition, as revealed by the symptoms, depend our subsequent action in the further treatment of the case.

The first thing to be determined is whether the remedy has acted at all or not. If it has not acted, we have next to determine whether the failure to act is due to an error in the selection of the remedy, or to the selection of the wrong potency of the remedy. If, in carefully reviewing our symptom-record, we find the remedy rightly chosen, we change the potency to a higher or lower potency, as circumstances may require, after a reconsideration of the patient's degree of susceptibility.

In deciding the question whether the remedy has acted or not, we must be careful not to be misled by the opinions or prejudices of the patient or his attendants. Some patients, having all their interest and attention centered upon some particular symptom which they regard as all-important, will assert that there has been no change; that they are no better, or even worse than they were before they took the remedy. These statements should be received with great caution and we should proceed to go over the symptom-record item by item with care. We need not antagonize the patient by gruffly asserting that he must be mistaken, but may express our regret or sympathy and then quietly question him as to each particular symptom. We will frequently find that the patient has really improved in many important respects, although his pet symptom (often constipation) is as yet unchanged.

The action of a remedy is shown by changes in the symptoms of the patient. Upon the character of those changes depends our further course of action. A remedy shows its action, 1. by producing new symptoms; 2. by the disappearance of symptoms; 3. by the increase or aggravation of symptoms; 4. by the amelioration of symptoms; 5. by a change in the order and direction of symptoms.

1. An improperly chosen remedy may change the condition of an oversensitive patient by producing new symptoms not related to the disease and detrimental to his welfare. These are pathogenetic symptoms. Their appearance indicates that the remedy is not curing the patient, but merely making a proving. Discontinuance and an antidote is demanded.

2. A correctly chosen remedy given in too low or sometimes too high a potency, or in too many doses, may cause an aggravation of the existing symptoms so severe as to endanger the life of the patient; especially if the patient be a child or a sensitive person and if a vital organ, like the brain or lungs be affected. Belladonna in the third or sixth potency, given in too frequent doses in a case of meningitis, for example, may cause death from overaction; whereas the thirtieth or two hundredth potency given in a single dose, or in doses repeated only until some change of symptoms is noticed, will speedily cure. Phosphorus 3rd or 6th in pneumonia under similar circumstances may rapidly cause death. The low potencies of deeply acting medicines are dangerous in such cases in proportion to their similarity to the symptoms.

The more accurate the selection of the medicine, the greater must be the care exercised not to injure the patient by prescribing potencies too low and doses too numerous. Medication should be stopped on the first appearance of such aggravations. An antidote should be administered if they do not speedily diminish. The careless prescriber rarely recognizes such aggravations. When he notices the symptoms he usually attributes them to the natural course of the disease or calls it a "complication."

3. A slight aggravation or intensification of the symptoms, appearing quickly after giving the remedy and soon passing away is a good sign. It calls for a suspension of medication until the after-following improvement ceases or the symptoms change again. It is the first and best evidence of the curative action of a well chosen remedy.

4. A prolonged aggravation without amelioration and with progressive decline of the patient is sometimes seen in chronic, deep seated disease as a result of the over-action of a deeply acting anti-psoric or anti-syphilitic medicine, given in too high a potency in the beginning of treatment. If the potency is too high its action may be too deep and far-reaching, and the reaction too great for the weakened vital power to carry on. Such remedies as Sulphur, Calcarea, Mercury, Arsenic and Phosphorus, given in the 50 M. or C.M., potencies, have sometimes hastened tubercular or tertiary syphilitic cases into the grave. In beginning treatment of suspicious or possibly incurable cases it is better to use medium potencies, like the 30th or 200th and go higher gradually, if necessary, as treatment progresses and the patient improves.

Very high potencies of the closely similar remedy are merciless searchers-out of hidden things. They will sometimes bring to light a veritable avalanche of symptoms which overwhelms the weakened patient. The disease has gone too far for such radical probing. If the disease has not gone so far, a long and severe aggravation may fortunately be followed by slow improvement. That patient was on the "borderland," with the beginning of serious destructive change in some vital organ.

In these homœopathic reactions and aggravations we distinguish between changes occurring in vital organs and changes in superficial tissues and non-vital organs. When old skin eruptions reappear, old ulcers break out again, old fistulæ re-open, old discharges flow again, swollen tubercular glands become inflamed, break down and suppurate away; old joint pains return; the patient's heart, lung, kidney, liver, spleen or brain symptoms in the meantime *improving;* then we know that both remedy and dose were right and a true cure is in progress. But if we find superficial symptoms disappearing and vital organs showing signs of advancing disease, we know we have failed.

The direction of cure is from within outward, from above downward and in the reverse order of the appearance of the symptoms. By this test we may always know whether we are curing or only palliating a disease. The last appearing symptoms of a disease should be the first to disappear under the action of a curative remedy.

In sub-acute and chronic diseases it is not unusual for preceding groups of symptoms to successively reappear as the later symptoms subside and cure progresses. This orderly change of symptoms should never be interfered with by repetition of doses nor change of remedy, so long as it continues. When improvement ceases or old symptoms reappear and remain without change it is time to repeat the dose.

5. The change following the administration of a remedy may be a *quick, short amelioration followed by a relapse to the original or a worse condition.* This may be because the remedy was only partly similar, or insufficient as to dosage; but where this occurrence is observed several times in succession and lasting improvement does not follow carefully selected remedies, it means that the case is incurable. There is not vitality enough to sustain a curative reaction, and dissolution is imminent.

6. In functional diseases, or in the beginning of acute organic diseases, accompanied perhaps by severe pain, the administration of the appropriate dose of the indicated remedy may be followed by rapid disappearance of symptoms without any aggravation. This is a cure of the most satisfactory kind, pleasing alike to physician and patient. Remedy and potency were both exactly right.

The Law of Dosage.—Summing up the matter, it appears that the law of dosage is contained in the law of similars, or the law of equivalents, both of which expressions are merely paraphrases of the law of Mutual Action, otherwise known as Newton's third law of motion.

The law might be stated thus: *The curative dose, like the remedy, must be similar in quantity and quality to the dose of the morbific agent which caused the disease.*

Von Grauvogl says:—"*The sole and simple question can only be what quantity of a substance is necessary, in order to induce that chemical or physical counter-motion in any diseased part of* the organism, which is equal in intensity, and opposite in direction, to that (motion) which is induced by the morbific cause, in order to check this latter forthwith, or at least to delay it, and then, by repetition, to remove it?" Stated in this form, the question conforms to the fundamental principle of homœopathy, *Similia Similibus Curantur,* which is a statement, in equivalent terms, of the third law of motion, *"action and reaction are equal and opposite."* Grauvogl goes on to state that "the task is only to discover the *equivalent of motion* between the amount of motion excited by the *morbid matter,* and the amount of motion which we have to oppose it by *some drug."* "For the solution of this problem," he says, "we have the natural law, according to which the *quality* contains the measure of the motion and the counter-motion; and hence, for the purpose of therapeutics, *the right dose must and can be nothing else than that amount of the indicated quality (or remedy) which is equal to the amount of the force of the cause of the disease, and qualitatively runs counter to its course and motions."* We possess thus, in the very dose, or *quantity of the morbid cause, the measure for the quantity of the dose of the drug to be used."* (And vice versa.)

At first sight, it might be objected that this leaves us as much in the dark as before, inasmuch as it does not indicate how we are to *measure the amount of force of the morbid cause.* But a little consideration will show that it does help us, because it suggests that *a measure may be found.* Perhaps a measure *has* been found. Let us see if this be not so.

Grauvogl is careful to warn us that we must not be misled into considering the *quality* of the external morbid cause as the measure of the dose, because the qualities of an external morbid agent, acting within the organism cannot be judged by quantities. A *quantity* or dose of a morbid substance so small as to be invisible, or imperceptible in any way except by its effects, might set up an action of such violent character in *quality* as to lead us to think the quantity must have been great. Under such circumstances the tendency and temptation is to give a remedy in doses the size and power of which correspond to our imagined dose of the morbid cause. In fact this is what is being done all the time, to the great injury of the human race. What violent and destructive actions are set up by the introduction into a wound of an infinitesimal quantity of septic matter from an imperfectly sterilized instrument! or by a single microscopic morbid cell or germ; or more remarkable still, by the influence of sudden violent emotion, purely mental and intangible as to quantity!

How then are we to measure these quantities?

The law of similars or equivalent actions reveals the answer, and mechanical potentiation according to scale gives the unit of measurement. The result is obtained by *simply reversing our rule of similars*. The real and efficient quantity of the morbid cause necessary to produce the disease *cannot be greater than the quantity of the medicine necessary to cure it!*

This conception, as a logical conclusion, enables us to put the matter upon an experimental basis and draw further conclusions as to the size of the dose. In this way we may test our low potencies, medium potencies, and high potencies, intelligently and logically.

Chemistry has given the clue to the mode of procedure in such cases, in its mode of determining the unit of measurement. Chemistry has established, with all the precision of a natural law, what quantity of acid, for example, is necessary to neutralize and saturate a given quantity of alkali.

The principle has thus been established in the abstract, but in a given case where the principle has to be practically applied, the chemist, like the homœopathic prescriber, must individualize, because he has often to deal with an unknown and undeterminate quantity.

Grauvogl illustrates it in this way: "No chemist," he says, "who wishes to ascertain how much potash a certain spring contains, would proceed as if he might assume a given quantity of potash empirically or traditionally, and forthwith add the quantity of acid corresponding thereto, necessary for saturation, to the given quantity of the mineral water; for, to say nothing about such a process as disregarding all the laws of the art of experiment, he must consider that, in dry seasons, all mineral waters are relatively richer in solid constituents than in wet seasons.

"He must, hence, begin with the *smallest* quantity of acid, highly diluted and add it, drop by drop, and count every drop till the experiment is concluded."

Precisely after the same rules of the art of experiment

might we proceed to find the dose in any particular case of disease. It may be said, however, that in subsequent examinations, the results of the first experiment might give a general point of departure from which an approximate determination of the necessary amount in similar cases could be had. Thus we might approximately determine, from a successful experiment with a certain potency of a remedy in a certain type of individual afflicted with a certain type of disease, the general value of that potency in its relation to similar conditions.

Actual experiments of this kind often upset preconceived notions, but the scientific man is always ready to bow to the logic of experience.

I was taught, for example, that "low potencies acted best in acute diseases." I accepted that generalization and acted upon it for some time before I discovered that it was altogether too broad, if not entirely false. It was not long before I witnessed a cure of an acute disease by a two hundredth potency so rapid and brilliant that I was encouraged to put it to the test myself. I succeeded in a number of cases and then I failed in a certain case. When I reflected upon the exception and sought for a reason why the high potency had acted in ten similar cases and failed in one, I found it in the grosser type of the individual and his lower degree of susceptibility, as well as in the lower grade of his disease process. He required a grosser, more material, lower form of a remedy to cure him.

I was taught also that infants and aged persons, being of low vitality and feeble reactive powers, required low potencies for their cure. Again I found that the generalization was altogether too broad; for I have cured the most desperate cases of croup, diphtheria, cholera infantum, etc., with a few doses of a high potency after they have been given up to die by those who had been prescribing tinctures and low potencies without avail; and I have seen as brilliant curative effects of high potencies in the aged as in the young, when both the remedy and the potency were indicated. Again we must individualize. Low potencies will not cure all acute diseases, all infants, nor all aged persons. Nor will high potencies cure all forms of disease in all persons. *All* potencies are required for the cure of disease, and *any* potency may be required in any given case.

CHAPTER XIV

Potentiation and the Infinitesimal Dose

Homœopathic potentiation is a mathematico-mechanical process for the reduction, according to scale, of crude, inert or poisonous medical substances to a state of physical solubility, physiological assimilability and therapeutic activity and harmlessness, for use as homœopathic healing remedies.

The primary object of potentiation is to reduce all substances designed for therapeutic use to "a state of approximately perfect solution or complete ionization, which is fully accomplished only by infinite dilution." (Arrhenius.) The greater the dilution, the higher the degree of ionization until, at infinite dilution, ionization is complete and therapeutic activity *conditionally* greatest.

For the reduction of minerals and inorganic substances and certain other substances, it employs mechanical trituration of one part of the substance with nine, or ninety-nine parts of pure crystalline sugar of milk, according as the decimal or centesimal scale of dilution is used. This process is continued long enough and in such a manner as to reduce them to an approximately impalpable powder, soluble in water. These, and all other soluble substances it reduces to liquids, or tinctures, which it still further reduces by dilution with water or alcohol in the same proportions of drug to vehicle (one to nine, or one to ninety-nine) to any degree determined upon, recording, numbering each step of the process in order that the degree of dilution and potentiation of each preparation may be known.

The resulting products of these operations are known as "potencies" or "dilutions," bearing the name of the medicine and the number of the dilution.

Originally all homœopathic remedies were prepared by hand, using the ancient and time honored mortar and pestle and the ordinary glass vial. Hand made potencies are still regarded by some as most reliable; but the products of time saving triturating and diluting machines, which have been invented and improved from time to time, are used by the majority of homœopathic pharmacists or potency makers.

By this process the most virulent and deadly poisons, even the serpent venoms, are not only rendered harmless, but are transformed into beneficent healing remedies. Substances which are medicinally inert in their crude natural state, such as the minerals, charcoal, or lycopodium, are thus rendered active and effective for healing the sick. Other drugs, more or less active in their natural state, have their medicinal qualities enhanced and their sphere of action broadened by being submitted to the process.

Arithmetical enumeration of the particles or proportions into which potentiation is supposed to divide a given quantity of the drug is insufficient and misleading. The facts go to show that the result of the process is not only a division of the matter into particles, *but a series of differentiations and progressions by which successive reproduction or propagations of the medical properties of the drug take place.* The powers and qualities of the drug are progressively transferred to the diluting medium. Recognizing this fact, Garth Wilkinson proposed to call them "transmissions."

Fincke explained the action and efficiency of infinitesimal doses by applying the "law of the least quantity," discovered by Maupertuis, the great French mathematician and accepted in science as a fundamental principle of the universe. That principle is stated as follows: *"the quantity of action necessary to effect any change in nature is the least possible."*

"According to this general principle," says Dr. Fincke, "the decisive moment is always a minimum, an infinitesimal." And to our therapeutics it will be perceived that the least possible is always the highest potency sufficient to bring about reaction and effect the cure, provided always that the selection of the remedy is homœopathically correct. "The Law of the Least Action *(Maxima Minimis)* appears to be an essential and necessary complement of the Law of Similars *(Similia Similibus)* and co-ordinate with it."

"According to this principle the curative properties and action of the homœopathic remedy are governed by its preparation and application; in other words, *the quality of the action of a homœo-*

pathic remedy is determined by its quantity. Consequently, the law of the least action must be acknowledged as the posological principle of homœopathy."

Potentiation and the minimum dose is a subject upon which it is exceedingly easy to form hasty and incorrect notions—no subject in homœopathy more so. It is one of those subjects upon which the average medical mind seems to have a peculiar natural bent for forming opinions without due knowledge and examination—in one word, prejudice. It may be said, however, that when the philosophy of homœopathy is understood, and its method of selecting the curative remedy has been mastered, decision as to the matter of the dose may be left safely to individual judgment, based upon observation and experience. The whole range of potencies is and should be open to every man. The beginner need be no more afraid of a thirtieth potency than of a third when he has decided upon the similar remedy; for he may be sure of this—*neither will cure if not indicated.* No one can make up his shortcomings as an accurate prescriber by increasing the size or frequency of his doses.

The idea of potentiation, or dynamization, as it is sometimes called, did not, like Minerva, spring "full armed and grown from her father's brain;" nor was the idea, like Minerva, "immediately admitted to the assembly of the gods." It was a gradual growth, a development. In some other respects, however, the idea *was* like Minerva. "The power of Minerva," we are told, "was great in heaven; she could hurl the thunders of Jupiter, *prolong the life of men, bestow the gift of prophecy and was the only one of all the divinities whose authority and consequence were equal to those of Jupiter."*

The greatest and keenest minds in homœopathy, the minds which have possessed insight in the highest degree, have always recognized the vital importance and fundamental relation of the doctrine of potentiation to homœopathy. It is at the same time the most vital and most vulnerable part, the very heart of homœopathy.

To quote only one of many authors, Prof. Samuel A. Jones of Ann Arbor: As long ago as 1872, when editor of the American Homœopathic Observer, he wrote these prophetic words, which have since been literally fulfilled. "Let us guard our homœopathic heritage most jealously. The provings on the healthy, the simillimum as the remedy, the single remedy, the *reduced* dose, may be and will be filched from us one by one and christened with new names to hide the theft. What will become of homœopathy? It will live, despite them, *in Hahnemann's posology*. The very infinitesimals which many are so ready to throw away are all that will save us."

This is only the recognition that, in its highest aspects, the doctrine *and the fact* of potentiation is one of those "mysteries of the faith" which have ever been the strength and at the same time the weakness, of every great church or school of thought; the strength because in their highest and broadest reaches they exercise the highest powers of the human mind; the weakest because they are the most liable to misunderstanding and perversion.

We may always rely upon our enemies to discover and attack the most vital and weakest part of our defenses. The proof of this statement lies in the fact that the doctrine of potentiation and the infinitesimal dose has always been the central point of attack upon homœopathy by its enemies.

Homœopathy was not created by the discovery of the law of similars. Many before Hahnemann, from Hippocrates down, had glimpses of the law, and some had tried to make use of it therapeutically; but all had failed because of their inability to properly graduate and adapt the dose. The principle of *similia* was of no practical use until the related principle of potentiation and the minimum dose was discovered; and that was not until Hahnemann, anticipating by a hundred years the modern conceptions of matter and force, hit upon the mathematico-mechanical expedient of preparing the drug by *dilution according to scale in a definite proportion of drug to inert vehicle*. Homœopathy became practicable at the moment that discovery was made and not before. But for that Hahnemann would have progressed no further than Hippocrates.

The tremendous scope and importance of his invention did not dawn upon Hahnemann at once. For a number of years in his original medical practice he had used drugs in the usual form and in ordinary doses. But as soon as he began applying medicine in such doses under the newly developed homœopathic principle, he found that aggravation and injury followed their use. Naturally this led him to reduce the size of the doses.

"Naturally," we say, although no one up to that time had ever thought of so simple and apparently obvious an expedient to overcome the obstacles to successful homœopathic practice. Finding that he obtained better results he continued to reduce the dose.

Hahnemann's idea at first was simply to reduce the "strength" or material mass of his drug, but his passion for accuracy led him to adopt a scale, that he might always be sure of the degree of reduction and establish a standard of comparison. Under certain conditions he found, perhaps to his surprise, that instead of weakening the drug he was actually increasing its curative power. In reducing the density of the mass he perceived that he was setting free powers previously latent, and that these powers were the greatest and most efficient for their therapeutic purposes, *when the remedy so prepared was applied under the principle of symptom similarity.*

Struck by the idea of the development of latent powers through what he had at first considered merely as dilution, he ceased calling the process "dilution," and named it "potentization" or "potentiation," which it truly is—a process of rendering potent, or powerful, that which was previously impotent.

Familiar to all is the trend of modern scientific thought away from the crudely materialistic notions of the early physical scientists, toward a higher conception of the constitution of matter.

Describing his conception of the nature and constitution of matter, Sir Isaac Newton quaintly said: "It seems probable to me that God in the beginning formed matter in *solid, massy, hard, impenetrable, movable particles,* of such sizes and figures, and with such other properties and in such proportion to space as most to conduce to the end for which he formed them; even *so very hard as never to wear or break in pieces;* no ordinary power being able to divide what God Himself made one in the first creation."

To Newton, light consisted of a perfect hail of these minute material atoms thrown off from the light producing body. In the exercise of his scientific imagination he saw these little particles of matter flying off in every direction at incredible speed.

Later came the conception of the luminiferous ether. Physicists think now of a ray of light as the pulsation or vibration of *an intangible substance which acts like a solid,* but which lets ordinary matter pass through it without interference.

The marvels of electricity as developed in such inventions as the dynamo, the electric motor, the electric light, the telegraph and telephone, and later the X-Ray and the wireless telegraph and radio, have done much to incline men toward the acceptance of a more spiritual interpretation of the universe. He who accepts without question the operations of this invisible, intangible force, the real nature of which no man knows, to say nothing of the phenomena of radio-activity, gravitation and chemical affinity, should not stumble over the homœopathic high potencies which he may make and demonstrate for himself any day.

Carl Snyder, in "New Conceptions in Science," points out how many advances in science and the arts have been made possible by the discovery of a *new mechanical appliance.* That homœopathy was thus made possible has not heretofore been recognized.

Snyder says:—"The phrase, 'mechanical appliance' is used broadly, as including all that may contribute to exact measurement and to the extension of our primitive senses in any direction. In this sense the calculus, or the reactions of the chemists testtube must be reckoned as mechanical no less than the thermometer, the microscope or the balance. It also includes such aids to calculation as the use of the zero (or more strictly speaking, a decimal system of counting); algebra, the inventions of fluxions, logarithms and the slide rule."

"We have all heard the story of how Archimedes detected the alloy in King Hiero's crown; how a certain weight of gold had been given by the King to an artificer to make over into a crown; how the King, suspecting a cheat, asked his friend Archimedes if he could tell whether base metal had been put in with gold; how Archimedes, sorely puzzled, stepped one day into his bath, observed how the water ran over, forgot everything and ran home naked through the streets of Syracuse shouting, Eureka! Eureka!"

"Archimedes' discovery was simply this; that a body in water **displaces** a quantity of water of *equal weight,* and not according

15

to its bulk, as one might believe at first thought. With it he established the idea of specific gravity.

By this he not only exposed the tricky goldsmith, but was led to all sorts of investigations, and finally to the discovery of the Lever."

In a similar way Hahnemann, groping about in his study of the action of homœopathic drugs on the healthy human organism, perplexed by the aggravations resulting from ordinary doses, seeking to find a dose so small that it would not endanger life and desiring to accurately measure his degree of dilution so that he might repeat or retrace his steps, invented or adopted *the centesimal scale of mensuration*. Immediately he found ready to his hand the means of solving the problem in which so many others before him had failed.

He had devised a process, simple in the extreme, by which, with nothing but a mortar and pestle, a series of small glass vials and a small quantity of sugar of milk, or of pure water or alcohol, he could not only modify toxic substances so that they were rendered harmless without destroying their curative powers, but develop and measure the inherent, latent medicinal energy of inert substances to any extent desired.

Substances which were entirely inert (physiologically or pathogenetically) in their natural state, such as the minerals, charcoal and lycopodium were by the newly invented process of trituration, solution and subsequent liquid potentiation, developed into medicines of remarkable power.

Homœopathy, as a practical art, thus became possible and Hahnemann passed on, leaving Hippocrates, Galen and all the other competitors in the race far behind.

And this was all brought about by the invention of a simple mathematical scale of measurements. It is so simple that only very few, even yet, begin to grasp its tremendous significance. One of the greatest physicists who ever lived, after reflection upon it, said that the Hahnemann theory of potentiation would ultimately lead to an entirely new conception of the constitution of matter. And so it has. Newton's "hard, massy, material atom" and even the atom of later physicists, is no more as an ultimate conception. It has given place to the immaterial electrical corpuscle, or electron, infinitely smaller and more active than the atom.

Historically, homœopathic potentiation is a development of very old and very common pharmaceutical processes. The mortar and pestle are as old as medicine. Minerals and inorganic substance are commonly prepared for therapeutic use by methods not only closely analogous, in its first stage, to the homœopathic method, but having their origin in the same fundamental necessity; namely, the necessity for rendering such substances soluble, capable of being taken up by the absorbents and appropriated by the sentient nerves of the living organism. Metals like mercury, lead and iron are entirely inert medicinally until they have been submitted to some process, physical or chemical, by which their mass is broken up and rendered soluble, and their latent medicinal energy thereby set free. It matters not by what name we call such a process, it is essentially a potentiation; and homœopathic potentiation is nothing more or less than *a physical process by which the dynamic energy, latent in crude substances, is liberated, developed and modified for use as medicines.*

Hahnemann, recognizing that the therapeutic action of a drug is the direct opposite of its physiological or toxic action, saw the possibility and necessity of extending this process, by perfectly simple, reliable and accurate means, so that it shall not only release the latent energy, but render it available for the higher purposes of healing by depriving it of its destructive or toxic action, while at the same time developing its purely therapeutic qualities and broadening its field of action.

It is perhaps not quite fair to imply that the dominant school has not recognized such a possibility. That it has done so is evidenced by its attempts to prepare certain morbid products, mostly of animal origin, for use as therapeutic agents by submitting them to a biological process which may be regarded as somewhat analogous to homœopathic potentiation. I refer to the processes by which the various serums and vaccines are prepared. The old time vaccination in which the patient was inoculated directly with the so-called "humanized" vaccine virus, represents its first attempt in this direction. So many evils arose from the practice that it was soon discontinued, and the more modern method devised. By this method, an animal, usually a calf, was inoculated with pus from a fully developed human smallpox pustule. After the ensuing disease thus set up in the animal had developed, serum or pus from one of the resulting pustules was again inoculated into another healthy animal to undergo the same or similar organic modifications. This process having been repeated a varying number of times, through a series of animals, the final product was used to inoculate human beings. With many technical modifications and extensions this is essentially the process used to-day in the preparation of the sera and vaccines.

The basic idea is to so modify a primarily virulent animal virus, toxin, or other pathological product, that it may be used safely for therapeutic or prophylactic purposes. In that respect it may be regarded as a crude analogue or imitation of homœopathic mechanical potentiation.

Considered as a technical process such a method is highly objectionable because it involves so many uncertainties. The living organism is an infinitely complex thing, when we consider the almost innumerable mechanical, chemical and vital processes going on within its constantly changing fluids and solids. Many of these processes are very imperfectly understood. There are no means of accurately registering and measuring all these activities; no means of determining exactly what these changes are; nor how they are modified by the introduction of the foreign morbid substance used.

In comparing this method with the Hahnemann process it is only necessary to point out:—

1. The Hahnemannian process is purely physical, objective and mechanical.

2. It does not involve any uncertain, unseen, unreliable nor unmeasurable factor. Its elements are simply the substance or drug to be potentiated, a vehicle consisting of sugar of milk, alcohol, or water, in certain quantities and definite proportions; manipulation under conditions which are entirely under control and so simple that a child could comply with them.

3. The resulting product is stable, or may easily be made so; in fact it is almost indestructible; and the experience of a century, in its use under homœopathic methods and principles has proved it

to be efficient and reliable in the treatment of all forms of disease amenable to medication.

4. The process is practically illimitable. Potentiation of medicine by this method may be carried to any extent desired or required.

To argue about a question which can be settled promptly by the actual test of experience is a waste of time and energy, for nothing is gained by it and we must come to the test of experience in the end. To rehearse the theories, speculations, mathematical computations, illustrations from analogy and comparisons with similar processes used in the allied arts and sciences, put forth by authors and disputants in discussing the pros and cons of the potentiation theory since it was first propounded by Hahnemann, might be interesting to some, but probably no one who has allowed himself to become prejudiced against homœopathic high potencies would be convinced by all the arguments thus stated.

But when a sincere investigator sees an expert examine and prescribe for a case under the methods and principles taught in the Organon and witnesses the therapeutic effects of the various potencies, he has seen a demonstration which he can repeat for himself until he is convinced that Hahnemann was right when he said; (par. 279) "Experience proves that the dose of a homœopathically selected remedy cannot be reduced so far as to be inferior in strength to the natural disease and to lose its power of extinguishing and curing at least a portion of the same, *provided that the dose, immediately after having been taken, is capable of causing a slight intensification of symptoms of the similar natural disease.*"

The results of the use of potentiated medicines have led careful students of the principles and conscientious practitioners of the methods of homœopathy, to gradually rise in the scale of potencies until many have come to use most frequently the higher potencies. This is because they are found to act more gently, more deeply, more rapidly and more thoroughly than the crude drug or the low dilutions, in the great majority of cases; and because it is impossible to cure certain forms of disease without them.

We have already seen how the idea of potentiation was made

practical by the invention of what was essentially a new mechanical appliance, the centesimal scale of mensuration, just as the mechanical performance of the mathematical processes of addition, subtraction, multiplication and division was made possible by the invention of the slide rule.

Unfortunately, when this discovery was first announced, attention was immediately focused upon the subject of *quantity* rather than upon *quality, proportionality and the laws of relation,* under which homœopathic medicines act. Objectors at once began to make arithmetical calculations of the *quantity* of the original drug to be found in the various potencies and to be staggered by the size of the denominators of the vulgar fractions which were supposed to express that quantity. To arithmetically express the fraction of the original drop of the "mother tincture" contained in one drop of the thirtieth centesimal potency requires a numerator of one, over a denominator of one, with sixty ciphers added!

That such an infinitesimal quantity of medicine could have any effect was for some, unthinkable. Thus, merely because of a seeming improbability, based upon *a priori* reasoning, without experiment, opposition to the new doctrine arose.

It never occurs to such minds to study the *laws of relation,* nor to ascertain experimentally whether such a potency really does act when brought into proper relations with the living organism. They refuse to submit it to the actual test of experience. To a scientific mind such an objection is not worthy of consideration. The objection of "improbability" in matters of fact is always childish. On such grounds every notable invention of the last century would be rejected. What more improbable than the assertion that a man, sitting in his office, could audibly converse with his friend three thousand miles away across the continent? But there stands the telephone on his desk ready for the demonstration.

The efficiency of homœopathic potencies is not to be determined by calculation, but by actual trial upon the living organism. If one desires to be convinced that there is power in the thirtieth potency of Arsenic, let him put ten drops of it in a half pint of water and begin taking tablespoonful doses of it every three hours. Convincing proof of its power will be experienced inside of three days.

To the mind of the mathematician, the astronomer, or the modern physicist, accustomed to think in the terms of the infinitesimal, such quantities present no difficulties, but to the unscientific mind, with its crude conception of the constitution of matter, they are unthinkable and incredible. It did not occur to the objectors to view the subject from the standpoint of *the laws of relation* under which such powers and quantities act, nor would their prejudices permit them to submit the matter to the simple test of practical experiment by which it could have been settled at once. Homœopathy, therefore, almost from the beginning, found its progress opposed by a prejudice based merely upon a seeming improbability.

The discovery of spectrum analysis, which revealed the presence of the drug as far as the twelfth centesimal potency, lent to the infinitely small quantities a significance not yet fully recognized in its bearing upon homœopathy; but even this, while it confirmed the *fact* of the presence of the drug, could not explain the *relation* of imponderable substances to the living organism.

The fact, as pointed out by Ozanam, is that Hahnemann, by his discovery of potentiation, raised homœopathy to a level with other natural sciences, since he created for it a method which is analogous to the infinitesimal calculus of mathematics, upon which is based the atomic theory of chemistry. It illustrates and harmonizes with the "theory of the interatomic ether of space;" the "theory of the radiant state of matter," the theory of the electric potential of present day physics, and with the chemico-cellular theory of physiology and pathological anatomy. It agrees with modern bacteriology in its explanation of the action of pathogenic micro-organisms as being due to the infinitesimal quantities of their secreted poisons. It is in harmony with the latest conclusions of modern psychology.

Von Grauvogl has shown that "the absorption of inorganic substances by the living organism regulates itself chiefly *according to the organic need,* hence such substances are taken into the organism only in very small quantities and in soluble form. Iron offers a good illustration. The physiological school found by experience that the natural Chalybeate springs were most efficacious in chlorotic-anæmic conditions, and yet the very strongest of these contains less than a grain of iron in sixteen ounces of water." In these later days, dependence is largely placed in so-called "organic iron" preparations derived from certain plants which contain very much less iron, and that existent in a highly vitalized or colloidal state.

A blood cell, among its other necessary constituents, contains a part or proportion of chloride of calcium which requires for its arithmetical expression a decimal of twenty-two places, corresponding to the eleventh centesimal potency. We are reminded by this of the remark of the celebrated physiologist, Valentin, who said; "The extreme minuteness and the immense quantity of the ultimate elements, everywhere engage our attention. The smallest image observable by the eye originates in millions of atmospheric vibrations. A grain of salt hardly large enough to taste, contains billions of groups of atoms, which no mortal eye can ever grasp. *Nature works everywhere with an infinite multitude of infinitely small magnitudes, which become appreciable to our comparatively dull senses in their ultimate masses only.*"

Baron Liebig, the celebrated chemist, denied and attempted to controvert homœopathic principles, especially the doctrine of potentiation, saying that it was absurd to suppose that decreasing quantity would increase efficiency. But when he found that common salt does not become suitable as a function remedy until attenuated in fifty times its own weight of water, he in fact potentiated it as Hahnemann did. Liebig contradicted himself many times on this subject in his writings. In his Chemical Letters, he says: "the heaviest manuring with the earthy phosphates and *coarse* powder can hardly be compared, in its effect, with a *far smaller quantity on a minutely divided state,* for, from this latter, we have the effect that a particle of manure is to be found in all parts of each small bit of soil. A single root-fibre requires *infinitely little* from the ground which it touches, but it is necessary, for its function and its existence, that this minimum *should be present at the very spot.*"

Even the soil itself can only receive and yield its chemical constituents in the form of a solution. As Liebig says, "If rain water, which contains ammonia, potash, phosphoric acid, silicic acid, in a state of solution, is brought into contact with the soil, then these substances leave the solution almost at once; the soil appropriates them from the water. If the soil did not possess this property, then these three chief nutritive substances *could not be kept in the earth."*

Thus, Liebig, the great opponent of homœopathy, gives involuntary testimony to the truth of the doctrine which specially excited his ire. Similar testimony abounds in all departments of science down to the present day.

The Relation of Inorganic Substances to the Living Organism.—Chemistry and physiology teach that many inorganic substances enter into the composition and structure of the living organism, and that the ordinary and normal source of these substances, as proximate principles, is the food and drink, and the air and light which we take to supply the processes of growth, nutrition and repair. These processes depend upon the vital functions of respiration, absorption, circulation, digestion, assimilation, secretion and excretion.

The inorganic elements or substances, with the exception of air, water and light, are not appropriated directly from the inorganic realm, but indirectly or mediately through the vegetable kingdom; or, once further removed, through the animal kingdom. The animal organism cannot assimilate inorganic substances in their natural state. They must first be modified; raised to a higher plane of existence, as it were; rendered more *similar* or assimilable to the substance of the animal organism, before they can be appropriated. In other words they must be *potentiated, dynamized* or *vitalized*—that is, raised to the plane of life by passing through the intermediate vegetable kingdom. Homœopathic potentiation is an artificial method of accomplishing this and for therapeutic purposes.

The living organism, vegetable or animal, can only assimilate that which is similar to itself, that is, similar to the elements of its own structure. The entire process of growth and assimilation, as it progresses from lower to higher forms, is simply *like appropriating like;* whether it be the blade of grass appropriating the molecule of silica, the ox appropriating the blade of grass, or man appropriating the flesh of ox in the form of juicy beefsteak. Even the blade of grass can only assimilate the silica in the form of silicic acid, which is practically silica dissolved in rain water! These processes represent natural physiological or organic potentiation. Air and light being imponderable, and water being fluid, or semi-ponderable, represent an intermediate scale of natural potencies. We can hardly call them high potencies, because there are so many other potencies in nature's realm of finer forces that are so much higher. They are high enough, or far enough removed from the grosser forms of inorganic substances, however, to be assimilable by the living organism and are rendered so by a sort of natural potentiation. We may get some idea of the relative importance of these degrees of potentiation to the living organism by recalling that a man may live forty days without food; he may live five to ten days without water, but he cannot live ten minutes without air.

Between each of the four realms of nature, mineral, vegetable, animal and spiritual, there is a chasm to be bridged; so that the representative organism of each realm consists of what might be called the machinery necessary for transforming the material of the next lower realm into the likeness of its own substance.

In all these transmissions, transformations and progressions the operation of the principle of *similia* is discernible. We also see the operation of the law of potentiation, for each step or degree of advance from a lower to a higher form or state of existence is, in reality, a potentiation—a development of the inherent powers and qualities of the elements. Under the transforming power of life in the blade of grass the inert molecule of silica is raised from the inorganic to the organic realm and *itself becomes living matter*. The forces which were latent in the inorganic become active and radiant in the organic. Gravitation, cohesion and chemical affinity, which held the silica in their grasp, yield to the chemistry of life. And so, when the succulent blade of grass is eaten, digested and assimilated by the sheep or the ox, or when the nourishing grain, or vegetable or fruit is assimilated by man; the process of transformation from the lower to the higher is always essentially a potentiation, ruled by similia and mediated by the infinitesimal. Thus, what we call "dead" or inanimate matter, by potentiation becomes living matter; for every particle of inorganic substance assimilated by the living organism is no longer dead but alive, and subject to the laws of life.

In a similar way, substances which in their natural state are unassimilable by the living organism, like the minerals, or substances which are toxic or destructive, are by homœopathic mechanical potentiation, rendered in the one case soluble, homogeneous and assimilable, and in the other case, not only harmless, but actually beneficent for the purpose of healing, when prescribed homœopathically. They become to the diseased organism what food is to the healthy organism; that is, reconstructive, in that they supply an organic need, restore order and harmony to disordered functions and permit a resumption of normal functioning.

The Scientific Foundation of Potentiation.—The researches of modern physical science have confirmed in a remarkable manner the century old teaching of Hahnemann in regard to the divisibility of matter and the power of the infinitesimal in medicine.

When Hahnemann first announced cures of disease by extremely small doses of medicine, his statements were received with incredulity and ridicule. Such a course of procedure was contrary to prevailing custom and belief. It did not avail to point out that the cures so effected were made by single remedies, instead of mixtures in common use; that the remedy for each case was selected under the guidance of a new principle in medicine; and that the remedies were prepared by a new process, by which their curative powers were conditionally greatly increased. Hahnemann's appeal to the medical profession to test the new method and publish results to the world was met by active opposition. He was forbidden to practice and was driven from his home by relentless persecution. The opposition begun at that time has never ceased, and the doctrine and practice have had to make their way against obstacles that would have been insurmountable to any but men who were firmly convinced that they were standing for a great and precious truth.

The use of the infinitesimal dose in homœopathy was the outcome of experience, but as a doctrine, it has its foundation in the truth embodied in the modern scientific theories of the conservation and energy and the indestructibility of matter.

In the doctrine of the *conservation of energy* physical science teaches that the sum total of the energy of the universe neither diminishes nor increases, though it may assume different forms successively. Physics, in the law of the *conservation of matter,* teaches that matter, as such, is indestructible and that the total quantity of it in the universe remains the same, regardless of the innumerable transformations and permutations constantly taking place in its component elements.

Mathematically, no limits can be assigned to the divisibility of matter. It is impossible to reach a division so fine as to be incapable of further sub-division. The smallest conceivable part will always contain *some* of the original substance and consequently some of its powers and qualities. It cannot possibly become *nothing.*

Practical experience with homœopathic high potencies in the treatment of the sick confirms these fundamental postulates of science. The highest potencies ever made by the Hahnemannian process of dilution, or by any modification of that process, have been shown to be capable of bringing about a curative reaction in the sick, when the remedy was homœopathic to the case.

Hahnemann taught, over a century ago, that *"the effect of a homœopathic dose is augmented by increasing the quantity of liquid in which the medicine is dissolved preparatory to its administration."* Recent scientific study of solutions, in working out in the laboratory the theory of *dissociation of molecules,* has verified the observation, and confirmed and amplified the theory of Hahnemann.

According to the later theory of the dissociation of molecules a chemical when dissolved is dissociated into parts smaller than the atoms of which it was composed. These particles are called ions. It has been proved that *the more dilute the solution, the greater the number of ions and the fewer the atoms. Complete ionization and absolute dissociation are possible only in infinite dilution.*

The following statement was made for the author by Mr. J. D. Burby, Chemist of the Electrical Testing Laboratories of New York.

"The theory of electrolytic dissociation or, simply, the ionization theory, was proposed in its completed form by Arrhenius to explain irregularities in the osmotic behavior of certain substances, notably inorganic acids, bases and salts. The theory is briefly that:—

"All substances belonging to the class which in water solution conduct electricity are, upon being dissolved in a dissociating solvent, dissociated into ions." Such substances are called electrolytes. It is to be particularly noted that the passage of an electric current through such a solution is not the cause of the dissociation, but rather, that dissociation takes place when the substance goes into solution, and it is because the solution contains the ions that it will conduct electricity.

Regarding the quantitative side of the theory, it need only be said that the degree of dissociation or ionization is a function of the dilution. The greater the dilution is the greater the degree of ionization, until at infinite dilution ionization is complete.

Further, the reactivity of electrolytes in dilute solution is measured by the degree to which they are ionized. Each substance has the property of dissociating to a definite extent when the solution has a certain concentration. Thus if equi-molecular solutions of hydrochloric, nitric, sulphuric and hydrofluoric acids are compared as regards the speed of reaction with a second substance, it will be found that the order in which they stand in this respect will be a measure of the degree to which they are ionized.

It would seem from this that the velocity of all reactions between electrolytes is greater, the greater the dilution and this is so with certain restrictions. Theoretically, the relative reactivity is greatest at infinite dilution because then the degree of ionization is greatest. Practically, however, there is a limit to this, because after a certain degree of dilution has been reached, the actual reactivity becomes too small to be of moment.

It should be further noted that the ionization theory applies particularly to inorganic acids, bases and salts, and that most organic compounds are very little dissociated, as we understand dissociation. Also, other solvents than water act as dissociating solvents, and among others may be mentioned liquid ammonia, liquid sulphur dioxide, and certain organic solvents."

In *chemistry* a molecule is defined as the smallest part of a compound substance that can exist separately and still retain its composition and properties; the smallest combination of atoms that will form a chemical compound.

In *physics,* the structural unity (molecule) is distinguished from the atom, and applied to particles of gases in the kinetic theory, independently of their relation to the chemical molecules.

Lord Kelvin illustrates the size of a molecule as follows:

"Imagine a rain drop or a globe of glass as large as a pea, to be magnified up to the size of the earth, each constituent molecule being magnified in the same proportion. The magnified structure would be coarser grained than a heap of small shot, but probably less coarse grained than a heap of cricket balls."

The smallest material thing in the world, the last in the series of little things known to modern science, is *the electron,* or electric corpuscle. It is supposed that the chemical atoms are composed of a collection of electrons having orbital motions in a sphere of positive electrification. The electron is conceived to be billions of times smaller than the atom. A French scientist compares the electrons in the atom to gnats in the dome of a cathedral.

It was formerly supposed that the atom was the smallest component part of matter. For a long time the atom had only a theoretical existence, its existence being assumed in order to account for the chemical combinations which take place between different elements in certain proportions. Even the ultra-microscope, which enables us to see and count particles of gold in ruby glass averaging six millionths of a millimeter in diameter, failed to reveal the atom. It remained for Rutherford, studying radium with his electroscope to identify and count individual atoms. Zeeman of Amsterdam, studying light through the spectroscope, split the spectral line of a flame, by holding the flame between the poles of a powerful electro-magnet, proving that light is an electric phenomenon, and showing a close relation between the activities of atoms and the origin of light itself.

Langley of the Smithsonian Institution invented *the bolometer,* which measures variations of temperature of one hundred millionth of a degree. This represents a change of temperature about equal to that produced by a candle five miles distant.

Light, traveling through space at the rate of 186,000 miles per second, has been found to *exert a distinct push or pressure.*

Hence, radiation, the force opposed to gravitation, must be considered in studying the movements of matter in a state of infinitesimal subdivision. This pressure force is measured by the radiometer, invented by two American physicists, Professors Nichols and Hull. It is used in connection with the bolometer, in measuring the rays from radio-active substances.

Pfund, of Johns Hopkins University, in 1913 perfected a still more sensitive instrument said to be capable of measuring a degree of heat equivalent to that given off by *a candle sixty miles away.*

Finally, ether, the all pervading, space filling entity, is regarded as something which is neither matter nor energy, but which serves as the medium through which both matter and energy are transmitted. Science regards the ether as an intangible or immaterial substance, which acts like a solid, but which allows ordinary matter to pass through it without resistance or disturbance. When it is caused to vibrate at a certain speed or rate it becomes visible as light. Light is defined as "an electro-magnetic disturbance of the ether." Ordinary light is defined as "the result of electric oscillation (or vibration) in the molecules or atoms of hot bodies, or sometimes of bodies not hot—as in the phenomena of phosphorescence."

Sir Oliver Lodge says, "the waves of light are not anything mechanical or material, but are something electrical and magnetic —they are, in fact, electrical disturbances periodic in space and time, and traveling with a known and tremendous speed through the ether of space. Their very existence depends upon the ether, their speed of propagation is its best known quantitative property."

Speaking of the ether, Lodge says:—"the ether has not yet been brought under the domain of simple mechanics—it has not yet been reduced to motion and force, and that probably because the *force* aspect of it has been so singularly elusive that it is a question whether we ought to think of it as material at all." * * * "Undoubtedly, the ether belongs to the material or physical universe, but it is not ordinary matter. I should prefer to say it is not 'matter' at all. It may be the *substance* or substratum, or *material of which matter is composed* but it would be confusing and inconvenient not to be able to discriminate between matter on the one hand and ether on the other." He further says,—"we do not yet know what electricity is, or what the ether is. We have as yet no dynamical explanation of either of them; but the past century has taught us what seems to their student an overwhelming quantity of facts about them. And when the present century, or the century after, lets us deeper into their secrets, and into the secrets of some other phenomena now in course of being rationally investigated, I feel as if it would be no merely material prospect that will be opening on our view, but some glimpse into a region of the universe which science has never entered yet, but which has been sought from far, and perhaps blindly apprehended, by painter and poet, by philosopher and saint." (Lodge—The Ether of Space.)

As a summary of present knowledge, Sir Oliver defines the ether of space as "a continuous, incompressible, stationary, *fundamental substance* or perfect fluid with what is equivalent to an inertia-coefficient of 10^{12} grammes per c.c.; that *matter* is composed of *modified and electrified specks, or minute structures of ether,* which are amenable to mechanical as well as to electrical force and add to the optical or electric density of the medium; and that elastic-rigidity and *all potential energy are due to excessively fine grained ethereal circulation,* with an intrinsic kinetic energy of the order 10^{33} ergs per cubic centimeter."

A. Wilford Hall, Ph.D., LL.D., Founder of the Substantial Philosophy, in The Problem of Human Life, had proved logically as early as 1875, that all the fundamental forces of the universe, including life, electricity and the ether of space are *substantial entities,* incorporeal, intangible and invisible, but capable of being perceived, measured and weighed.

Modern science has practically accepted this conclusion, for today we have Sir Oliver Lodge, the greatest living correlator and interpreter of the facts of science, defining the ether of space as the most tenuous and refined *substance* known to science, and submitting mathematical computations of its physical properties.

Having anticipated the theory and conclusions of the chemist and physicist by clinical experience with high potencies in the treatment of the sick, the followers of Hahnemann are in a position to maintain, with authority, that the curative power of a drug is not lost when it is diluted to such a degree that a dose represents an amount of actual drug substance so small as to be practically an unassignable quantity—in other words, an infinitesimal quantity.

But the doctrine of Potentiation and the Infinitesimal Dose has another important application in medicine.

Fincke (On High Potencies) says: "Disease originates in the specific action of noxious matter which is either produced within the organism, or brought in from without, and it is always carried on by a process of assimilation."

"Assimilation, everywhere, is accompanied by *potentiation*, by rendering the infinitesimal particles of matter susceptible and active, according to their inherent affinities."

"As homœopathic remedies are obtained by potentiation, that is by comminuting and refining drug matter, by means of a vehicle easily assimilable; so nutritious matter appears to stand (act) as the vehicle in the *natural potentiation* of those noxious materials which the organism itself prepares as remedies for its own self-preservation" (antitoxins, antibodies, etc.).

"As the whole organism draws upon digestion, as the source of its nutrition, so every part and particle of the organism draws upon the various materials successively worked out by the different processes of animal chemistry for its own proper nutriment, and assimilates them for its own particular use and subsistence. Thus, the lacteals draw upon the chyle prepared by digestion; the lymphatics upon the transudation of the capillaries, the blood upon the fluids of either of these; and the nerves upon the blood."

"Those parts of the organism which do not satisfy their wants and requirements by this intra-organic nutrition alone, assimilate from the outer world whatever is necessary, not only for their own existence, but also for their co-operation with others and for the self-preservation of the organism. Thus the blood assimilates oxygen from the air; the eye, light; the ear, sound; the nose, olfactory matter; the tongue, gustatory matter; the brain and nerves, phosphorus, etc.; the mind (thought or) the operations of other minds by means of the senses, and so on; the organism continually assimilating from the Planet and the Universe as long as it lasts. Consequently the whole organism is the product of assimilation of matter, *and its action is the result of potentiation of matter*. And so is disease. And so is health. And so is all life."

"The hypothetical ether is, possibly, *infinitesimal comminuted matter,* forming, as it were, *the reservoir of the high potencies required for the Universal Assimilation or Homœosis,* which is continually going on and mediating all life in the world."

These words were written prior to 1865—more than fifty years ago. Does it not increase our respect and reverence for our Dr. Fincke as a philosopher to find Sir Oliver Lodge, the foremost philosopher and scientist of Great Britain, substantially endorsing his views in his work, "The Ether of Space," published in 1909?

Lodge says:—"The question is often asked, is ether material? This is largely a question of words and convenience. Undoubtedly, the ether belongs to the material or physical universe, but it is not ordinary matter. I should prefer to say it is not "matter" at all. It may be the *substance* or substratum of material of which matter is composed, but it would be confusing and inconvenient not to be able to discriminate between matter on the one hand and ether on the other. If you tie a knot on a bit of string, the knot is composed of string, but the string is not composed of knots. If you have a smoke or vortex ring in the air, the vortex ring is made of air, but the atmosphere is not a vortex ring.

"The essential distinction between matter and ether is that matter *moves,* in the sense that it has the property of locomotion and can effect impact and bombardment; while ether is *strained* and has the property of exerting stress and recoil. All potential energy exists in the ether. It may vibrate and it may rotate, but as regards locomotion it is stationary—the most stationary body we know; absolutely stationary, so to speak; our standard of rest. All that we ourselves can effect, in the material universe, is to alter the motion and configuration of masses of matter. * * *

"But now comes the question. How is it possible for matter to be composed of ether? How is it possible for a solid to be made out of a fluid? A solid possesses the properties of rigidity, impenetrability, elasticity, and such like; how can these be imitated by a perfect fluid such as the ether must be?"

The answer is, They can be imitated by *a fluid in motion;* a statement which we make with confidence as the result of a great part of Lord Kelvin's work.

"It may be illustrated by a few experiments."

"A wheel of spokes, transparent or permeable when stationary, becomes opaque when revolving, so that a ball thrown against it does not go through but rebounds. The motion only affects permeability to matter; transparency to light is unaffected."

"A flexible chain, set spinning, can stand up on end while the motion continues."

"A jet of water at sufficient speed can be struck with a hammer and resists being cut with a sword." * * *

"If ether can be set spinning, therefore, we have some hope of making it imitate the properties of matter, or even of constructing matter by its aid. But *how* are we to spin the ether? Matter alone seems to have no grip on it." * * *

"But you can vibrate it electrically; and every source of radiation does that. An electrical charge, in sufficiently rapid vibration, is the only source of ether waves that we know; and if an electric charge is suddenly stopped, it generates the pulses known as X-Rays, as the result of the collision. Not speed, but sudden change of speed is the necessary condition for generating waves in the ether by electricity." * * *

"The universe we are living in is an extraordinary one, and our investigation of it has only just begun. We know that matter has a psychical significance, since it can constitute *brain*, which links together the physical and psychical worlds. If any one thinks that the ether, with all its massiveness and energy, has probably no psychical significance, I find myself unable to agree with him."

"The earliest conception of ether regarded it as simply a medium for conveying radiation. Faraday's experiments and investigations led him to believe that it had other perhaps more important uses and properties. He conjectured that the same medium which is concerned in the propagation of light might also be the agent in electromagnetic phenomena, and this conjecture was amply strengthened by subsequent investigations."

Lodge now says:—"One more function is now being discovered; *the ether is being found to constitute matter.*"

Prof. Sir J. J. Thomson says:—"The *whole* mass of any body is just the mass of ether surrounding the body which is carried along by the Faraday tubes associated with the atoms of the body. *In fact, all mass is mass of the ether; all momentum,*

momentum of the ether and all kinetic energy, kinetic energy of the ether." This view, it should be said, requires the density of the ether to be immensely greater than that of any known substance."

Thus we see that the difference between Dr. Fincke's conception of the constitution of the ether and that of Faraday and the later scientists is mainly verbal. There is no appreciable difference between the ether as "matter in a state of *infinitesimal fineness of division,*" and the ether as the "substance of which matter is composed." Comprehension of either idea depends upon the ability to understand the meaning of the word infinitesimal as used in the mathematical sense. "Infinitely small," denotes a quantity conceived as continually diminishing so as to become *less* than any other quantity having an assigned value. There is no limit assigned nor conceivable. It is finite thought carried to the utmost limit "and then some."

The philosopher, the physicist and chemist, each in his own way, analyzes, divides and subdivides matter until he can go no farther, and then finds himself confronted by a mystery, incapable of solution by physical means. Shall he stop there and hush the question that will arise in his mind when he has penetrated thus far? Something within him rebels at the arbitrary limitation of thought. Aspiration, intuition, reason, analogy, the logical faculty, all urge him forward. Up to this point his investigation has revealed what can only be regarded logically as secondary causes. The primary cause eludes him. The physician and pathologist also has his mystery. The microbe, the bacillus, the bacterium, all forms of micro-organisms and all other proximate causes of disease, carried back even to the formless bit of protoplasm or living matter, must themselves be accounted for. That which lies beyond cannot be seen by the microscope. At this point, it is necessary to substitute the telescope of intuitional reasoning for the microscope of physical demonstration.

CHAPTER XV

The Drug Potential

The homœopathic theory of drug potentiation may be considered as an extension into medicine of what is known in physical science as the "Theory of the Potential," a function of fundamental importance in the Theory of Attractions, under which the greater part of the modern progress in invention has been made.

To give Hahnemann his just dues as an original investigator in science, however, and to place his dynamical theory in its right relation to modern scientific thought, it should be remembered that he promulgated his theory of potentiation long before the Theory of the Potential was announced. It was pointed out even during Hahnemann's lifetime that his experiments and the theory based upon them opened the way for an entirely new consideration of the subject of dynamics, and led to new conceptions of the constitution of matter. It would be permissible, therefore, from the chronological standpoint, to reverse the opening statement of this article and say that the modern scientific Theory of the Potential is an extension into physics of Hahnemann's pharmaco-dynamical Theory of Potentiation.

For the clearest and most concise definition of the Theory of the Potential I quote the Standard Dictionary:

"Potential exists by virtue of position, as opposed to motion; said especially of energy."

1. Potential is a condition at a point in space, due to attraction or repulsion near it, in virtue of which something at that point, as a mass or electric charge, would possess potential energy or the power of doing work; in the case of electricity, measured by the work done in bringing a unit of positive electricity thither from an infinite distance against an electrical repulsive force.

2. In any system of attracting bodies, a mathematical quantity having at each point of space, a value equal to energy acquired by a unit mass in falling from an infinite distance to that point.

Potential, regarded as something distributed throughout space, determines, by the difference of its values at neighboring points, the intensity and direction of the force acting through the region. Its variation from one point to another thus constitutes or at least measures force, the law being that a material body always tends to move in the direction of increasing potential and a positive electrical charge in that of decreasing potential. The function in the former case is called *gravitation potential*, and in the latter *electrical potential*, which is taken from the opposite algebraic sign.

Electrical potential, which determines the flow of electricity, has been compared to *temperature*, which similarly governs the flow of heat. The potential due to the earth's attraction in like manner determines *level*, which governs the flow of water."

To this we may now perhaps add that the *drug potential*, due to the attraction of the living organism, determines, in a similar manner, the direction and kind of action of the drug prescribed or taken.

Have we not here suggested in this contribution from an allied science, a possible means of measuring the power and action of infinitesimal doses of medicine in the living organism? In physiological experimentation we have to deal with the living organism, energized by a power which exerts a force akin to, if not identical with, electricity—but one which, in its physical manifestations, is demonstrably governed by the laws of motion. That force should be measurable by the methods and standards used in physical science.

Here is a suggestion for our research workers. Let them lay aside for a time their unfruitful studies of serums, vaccines and micro-organisms, and devote their attention to the subject of vital energy as manifested in living organisms. Let them learn how to measure the actions and reactions of that fundamental, entitative power and principle called Life in the same way that the electrical scientist measures the force with which he deals in his department.

The idea of a drug potential, analogous to the electrical and gravitation potential, has never been advanced before, as far as

I know; but it appears to be one capable of being worked out mathematically by some one who is competent. It is merely presented here as a suggestion which may lead to the discovery of a new means of measuring the dynamic energy and mode of action of potentiated homœopathic medicines.

Something determines the intensity and direction of the force of a drug acting within its sphere in the living organism; and its variation from one point to another, or from one condition or state to another, might be made to mathematically measure its force, if such a measurement were desirable for any purpose.

Does a crude drug in massive dose act under the same law as a material body and tend to move in the direction of increasing potential? And does an infinitesimal dose obey the law which makes a positive electrical charge tend to move in the opposite direction toward a decreasing potential, and thus effect cure of disease? We know that the direction of action of the massive dose is opposite to the action of the infinitesimal dose, as we know that the direction of the organic forces of health is opposite to that of disease.

We know that a peculiar affinity or attraction exists between a sick organism and the drug which is capable of producing symptoms in a healthy organism similar to those of the sickness.

The theory of the symptomatically similar medicine as a curative is, therefore, also "a phase of the theory of attractions," of which the theory of the potential is another phase.

A dose of medicine placed on the tongue, in contact with the sentient nerves of the organism, from which it is distributed throughout the entire nervous system, is a "something at the point in space at which there exists a condition of attraction or repulsion caused by its presence there." The dose, according to its size and quality, may be a "mass," or it may be an "ion," an infinitesimal dynamic quantity, comparable to "an electric charge."

The action of a drug upon the living substance is analagous to the action of electricity and has often been compared to it. There are some who even believe that life and electricity are identical.

When Hahnemann adopted the plan of proving drugs on the healthy and thus brought drug action within the category of observable phenomena, he opened up a new field in physical science and made possible the formation of a dynamical theory, by which their action may not only be physically explained, but measured, modified and controlled.

In the scientific sense, then, we say that Hahnemann, through drug-proving and potentiation, was enabled to formulate a dynamical theory, and raise materia medica to the level of a science. In other words, he might be said to have discovered the *drug potential,* and brought materia medica and therapeutics into alignment with the other sciences which are based upon the theory of the potential.

The Hahnemannian theory and process of potentiation makes it possible to modify and govern, as well as to measure, the action of drugs submitted to proving, or prescribed under the principle of *similia,* to any extent required. As the development of the modern sciences of electricity, hydrostatics, and engineering has been due largely to the application of the theory of the potential, so has the development of homœopathy been due to the application of a similar theory in medicine.

The theory of the drug potential appears to be a logical corollary of the dynamical theory of life, the law of similars and the law of potentiation. Taken together they make up the great triad of fundamental principles in the Hahnemannian philosophy. If we view life from the standpoint of dynamics, considering health as orderly, balanced and harmonious action and disease as unbalanced or disorderly action of the life principle, then we must also consider the agents which change or modify the action of the life principle from the same standpoint. Any agent or substance which modifies the action of the life principle medicinally must do so by virtue of its inherent dynamic energy; and that action must be governed fundamentally by the same dynamical laws which govern the operation of the life principle physiologically and pathologically.

These laws are related to all the vital functions, and to all the agents which act upon and modify them. The organs of nutrition, growth and repair; digestion, absorption and excretion; innervation and enervation; respiration, circulation, sleep; intellect, emotion, memory, reason, judgment and will all react to appropriate stimuli under the law of attraction and mutual action, stated by Sir Isaac Newton in the formula, "action and reaction are equal and opposite."

These same laws, in the last analysis, govern all the agents and substances which act upon the living organism. They are related to the germination, growth and reproduction, and the development of the inherent properties of all the plants and forms of vegetable life from which we derive our drugs; to the functional and organic development and existence of all the insects, reptiles, and other forms of animal life which furnish their secretions for our medicinal use; and to the origin, formation and constitution of all the minerals and inorganic substances which make up a part of our materia medica. The embodied dynamic energy of each and all of these becomes available and useful through Hahnemann's discovery of the drug potential and his invention of the mechanical process of homœopathic potentiation.

The form or manner in which the dynamic energy of any particular substance manifests itself depends upon its physical condition, and upon the condition of the organism in which it acts.

The knowledge that drugs act upon the living organism, and that the organism reacts to drugs; and the further knowledge that the organism reacts in a different manner to each drug, led to the recognition of the specific character of drug action and to the doctrine of elective affinities; that each drug had a specific or peculiar relation to or affinity for the living organism, differing from the action of every other drug.

Prior to Hahnemann's time, with only a very few exceptions, this idea was limited in its application to diseased conditions alone. Drugs were used to modify diseased conditions upon fanciful or theoretical grounds, without any knowledge of their action upon the healthy organism. Empiricism reigned in medicine. Deluded and hampered by the idea that disease was an entity, the futile search for specifics for *diseases* began, and has continued to this day, regardless of the obvious fact that no two persons affected with the same disease are affected in exactly the same manner, and that, therefore, there can be no such thing as a specific for a disease. Disease is not an entity but a process—a constantly changing condition or state.

The doctrine of specifics applies to disease as well as to drugs, but it is limited to the *individual*. It does not apply to the class. The direct, producing causes of disease are entities, but the cause can only become active under certain conditions, and the action of any disease-producing substance is always modified by the peculiar character and conditions of the individual and his environment. This modification must always be taken into consideration in practice. The practical problem is to find the remedy for the individual and correctly measure its power and action.

Hahnemann attacked the problem from a new standpoint when he began to investigate the action of drugs upon the *healthy* human organism. By his tests or "provings" he showed that the healthy organism has an attraction for drugs and that it will react to their influence, under proper conditions, in the production of objective and subjective phenomena, or symptoms. By observing these phenomena the peculiar or specific properties and character of drugs may be definitely determined and measured. Drug action is thus proven to be dynamical and brought within the scope of the general law of attraction.

Knowledge of the existence of this attraction or affinity of the living organism for drugs and of the phenomena which they produce, taken with the conditions under which they are produced, opens the way for the formulation of a dynamical theory of how they act. The power which they exert, or the power which the organism exerts in reacting to them may be both measured and controlled. Considered from the standpoint of dynamics we have here *quantities* with which to deal, the same as in any other department of physics. Power of a specific kind is generated, applied and expended for a specific purpose—drug or medicinal power for proving or cure. The drug possesses potential energy, or the power of doing work of a certain kind in the living organism, under certain conditions. The quantities dealt with are assignable quantities and may be measured mathematically or otherwise.

Hahnemann's first great discovery was that *the quality of the drug action is governed by the quantity of the drug used.*

In order to control drug action, therefore, it was necessary to find and adopt a scale of mensuration for drugs which should be both quantitative and qualitative. The centesimal scale of dilution adopted by Hahnemann practically fulfills the requirements for quantitative measurement of drug action and satisfies the pure therapeutist even as a qualitative yardstick; but for the scientist it leaves something to be desired in accuracy for qualitative measurement.

It remains true, however, that Hahnemann's conception of the dynamic nature of drug and disease action brought their phenomena within the scope of the universal laws of motion and made possible the development of an efficient system of therapeutic medication.

CHAPTER XVI

The Logic of Homœopathy

The logical principles which underlie homœopathic prescribing are commonly overlooked. Apparently there are almost as many methods of prescribing as there are prescribers. The remarkable cures performed by such men as Bönninghausen, Lippe, Dunham and Wells are commonly regarded as having been due to some mysterious power possessed by them as individuals. That similar results are attainable by anyone who will master the method is difficult for many to believe; yet a clear and comprehensive statement of the principles involved and an identification of the source from which they are drawn will be sought in vain in homœopathic literature.

As a rule, only personal opinions and fragmentary statements by individuals of how they did or thought they did their prescribing will be found, and these are scattered through a voluminous literature, much of which is out of print and difficult of access. They indicate, however, that there is a basic method somewhere, if only it can be found and identified.

Reviewing these collected bits of personal teaching and experience creates an impression that their authors were either unaware, perhaps through forgetfulness, of the nature of the principles they were using; or that they took it for granted that the student already possessed the requisite knowledge. They did not seem to realize the educational value and importance to the student of being able to identify and consciously use an unnamed science which is fundamentally related to medicine, and especially to homœopathy; for they certainly did not name it, nor definitely refer to it. This is not so strange or unusual as it may seem.

Monsieur Jourdain, an amusing character in one of Moliere's plays, expressed great surprise on learning that he had been *talking prose* for more than forty years.

"Ninety-nine people out of a hundred," says Jevons, "might be equally surprised on learning that they had long been converting propositions, syllogizing, falling into paralogisms, framing hypotheses and making classifications with genera and species. If asked whether they were logicians they would probably answer, No! They would be partly right; for I believe that a large number even of educated persons, have no clear idea of what logic is. Yet, in a certain way, everyone must have been a logician since he began to speak. * * * All people are logicians in some manner or degree; but unfortunately many persons are bad ones, and suffer harm in consequence." Hence the necessity of books and essays on logic.

It is equally true that ninety-nine homœopathic physicians out of a hundred might be surprised on learning that they had been using logic, good or bad, in every prescription they ever made.

They might be still more surprised on learning that homœopathy itself is founded and constructed upon logical principles; and that all its processes may, and if they are to be correctly and efficiently performed must, be conducted under the principles and by the methods of good logic.

It was very stupid of me, of course, but I had been practicing homœopathy a good many years and making, I thought, some pretty good prescriptions, before it dawned upon me in any definite way that logic as a science had any technical connection with homœopathic prescribing. It was a "purple moment" for me when I made that discovery. It explained all my good prescriptions and accounted for all my bad ones which, of course, outnumbered the good ones ten to one. It opened up possibilities of improving my methods and bringing the percentage of cures a little more in my favor. If the making of a good prescription, a good examination, or a good diagnosis depended upon a correct application of the principles of logic, I saw that it behooved me to get down my old textbooks on logic, long before relegated to an upper shelf in my library, along with certain other old school books which some of us like to preserve for sentimental reasons, and refresh my memory by a review of the subject in the light of experience.

It also occurred to me to examine into the mental processes

of acknowledged masters of the art of homœopathic prescribing from that point of view and try to make out how they did it.

It is surprising how such a middle-age review of one's youthful studies will sometimes dispel delusions long fondly held.

How many, for example, recall and realize the practical bearing of the fact that the science of logic exists in two parts—the logic of form and the logic of reality or truth; or, technically, Pure or Formal Logic and Inductive Logic.

An outline of a few of the principal operations of formal logic is about all most of us can recall in any definite way. Our ordinary mental processes are governed largely by what was hammered into us in youth. If we try to analyze our mental processes we are likely to think in the terms of formal logic, because formal logic is what is usually taught, and formal logic is what sticks.

Now formal logic, with all its fascinating processes, takes no account of *the matter* of our reasonings—of the things reasoned about. Formal logic deals solely with the form, or skeleton of the *reasoning itself*. It does not concern itself in the least with the truth or falsity of a statement as a matter of fact or science. Its purpose is to provide the general or symbolic forms which reasoning must assume in order to insure that the end of a proposition may be consistent with its beginning. Its object is merely consistency, and "consistency's a jewel" of sometimes doubtful value. Emerson wittily said: "A foolish consistency is the hobgoblin of little minds." So there may be a *foolish consistency* as well as a *false logic*. A rogue may be as good a logician as an honest man—perhaps a better; a quack may be as logical as the most ethical practitioner; and an allopath, who gives his massive doses of combined drugs upon empirical grounds, may be as consistent, from the standpoint of formal logic, as the homœopath who gives only minimum doses of the single, similar remedy.

Each of these can and does take his stand against the world, on the ground that he is logical and consistent. His conclusions are consistent with his premises; and there you have the psychology of it, with the secret of the arrogance of the average medical man.

"He was in Logic a great critic,
    Profoundly skilled in analytic;
  He could distinguish and divide
  A hair "twixt the south and southwest side."

He does not know, nor wish to know what some of us may have learned and forgotten—that *Inductive Logic,* the Logic of Bacon, Mill and Hahnemann, has a higher function than the Logic of Aristotle, which exists and is used largely for the purpose of mere argumentation.

Inductive Logic *does* concern itself with facts, with reality. Its primary purpose is the discovery and use of *Truth.*

The first requirement of Inductive Logic is that *the premises must be true,* the result of true and valid observation of facts, based, if need be, upon pure experimentation.

Before we proceed to make deductions, classifications and generalizations and spin theories, we must be sure that we have reliable facts. The induction must be complete, without break, from premise to conclusion. We may not reason from a hypothesis, nor jump to a conclusion, as medical sophists do. We must follow the course laid down, and "keep in the middle of the road." The road into the great unknown is dark and full of pitfalls for the unwary, but the electric lamp of inductive logic lights the way safely from the known into the unknown.

This is *The Logic of Homœopathy.* This is what we mean when we say that homœopathy is based upon the inductive philosophy. Not only are the conclusions of homœopathy consistent with its premises, but its premises are founded upon Truth; for homœopathy as a method is drawn logically, according to the strictest rules of inductive generalization, from data which have been derived from direct observation of facts and pure experimentation. Every one of its processes, from the conduct of the proving to the making of a curative prescription, is governed by the principles of inductive as well as deductive logic.

The purpose of this part of the work is not to instruct the reader in the elements of logic, but simply to define and discuss some of the more general relations of logic to the various processes of applied homœopathy; and to point out the great advantage that accrues to the physician who consciously and definitely uses the methods of inductive logic in his daily work.

If the reader's early education in formal logic has been deficient, it will be an easy matter for him to gain the requisite knowledge from any standard work on the subject.

The Inductive Method in Science is the application of the principles of inductive logic to scientific research. This method was originated by Lord Bacon, and set forth in his *Novum Organum*. It was further developed by John Stuart Will in his great *System of Logic*. It has been the inspiration, the basis and the instrument of every modern science.

Inductive Logic Defined.—"The Inductive Method in Logic is the scientific method that proceeds by induction. It requires (1) *exact observation;* (2) *correct interpretation* of the observed facts with a view to understanding them in relation to each other and to their causes; (3) *rational explanation* of the facts by referring them to their real cause or law; and (4) *scientific construction;* putting the facts in such co-ordination that the system reached shall agree with the reality."

"The search for the cause of anything may proceed according to any one of four methods: (1) the *method of agreement,* in which a condition uniformly present is assumed to be probably a cause; (2) the *method of difference,* in which the happening of an event when a condition is present, and its failure when a condition is absent, lead to the assumption of that condition as a cause; (3) the *method of concomitant variations,* in which the simultaneous variation in similar degree of condition and event establishes a casual relation; and (4) the *method of residues* or of residual variations, where after subtracting from a phenomenon the part due to causes already established the remainder is held to be due to some other unascertained cause or to the known remaining causes." (F. & W. Standard Dictionary.)

Before Lord Bacon's time, logic was used principally as an instrument for argument and disputation. Little or no attention was given to facts. Direct and systematic investigation of nature was unknown or ignored. Opinions, speculations and theories were used as the material for constructing more opinions and theories. The search for truth ended nowhere.

Lord Bacon called upon men to cease speculating and go direct to nature in their search for truth. He demolished innumerable false systems and restored logic to its true place as the guide to truth.

"There are and can exist," says Bacon, "but two ways of investigating and discovering truth. The one hurries on rapidly from the senses and particulars to the most general axioms; and from them as principles and their supposed indisputable truth derives and discovers the intermediate axioms. This is the way now in use. The other constructs its axioms from the senses and particulars, by ascending continually and gradually, till it finally arrives at the most general axioms, which is the true but unattempted way." (Nov. Org. Axiom 19.)

As induction is the antonym of deduction it has been supposed that the two processes are in some way antagonistic. This is an error. They are simply opposite ways of arriving at the same conclusions; two modes of using the same general process, namely: inference, or inferring.

All reasoning is inference, and in the last analysis all reasoning is deductive. By inductive reasoning we ascertain what is true of many different things. Our senses tell us what happens around us and by proper reasoning we may discover the laws of nature, in consequence of which they happen.

In deductive reasoning we do the opposite and infer what will happen in consequence of the laws.

Reasoning *a priori* and *a posteriori* are not different modes of reasoning, but arguments differing in the character of one of the premises. It is merely a difference of viewpoint. In one we reason from antecedents, in the other from consequents.

True says:—"Logic is the science of inference; it teaches how one judgment may be inferred from other judgments. To reason is to infer, hence it is usually called the science of reasoning."

"It assumes that every mind conceives intuitively some ideas or judgments which are at once primary and certain; otherwise we could have no foundation for inference; and to infer one idea or judgment from others would give no certainty."

"These ideas are called first truths. They are given by the senses, the consciousness and the reason, and they are innumerable. *I exist. There is an external world. This body is solid, extended, round, red, warm or cold,* are first truths."

"At first these ideas are particular, but afterward the mind unites those which are similar, or which agree in some respect, into classes. This is called generalization. To express this we no longer say this or that body, but body; not coat, shirt, trousers, etc.; but clothes."

To test their qualifications in this respect, I once gave a senior class of medical students a list of garments and asked them to generalize it: Only one man, in a class of about thirty, was able, off-hand, to reply correctly—"clothes!"

To show that all reasoning is, in the last analysis, deductive, True uses the following illustrations: "I infer that heat in such a degree as will cause the mercury in the thermometer to rise to the point marked two hundred and twelve degrees Fahrenheit *will always cause water to boil;* in other words, it is proved by induction to be a law of nature that two hundred and twelve degrees Fahrenheit will cause water to boil.

"Now the conclusion is not drawn from any number of instances of the boiling of water, but with a few instances combined with the principle *that like causes will produce like effects;* for if this principle were not true, then forty thousand instances of water boiling would not prove that another case would happen. But now I know like causes will produce like effects, and I know by observation that two hundred and twelve degrees Fahrenheit did once or twice cause water to boil. Admit the premises and the conclusion is unavoidable; and to do this is simply to affirm something of a class, then to refer the individual to that class, and then to affirm the same thing of the individual." "Now the first premise is the *general principle, which is intuitively true.* The only question is about the second premise; namely: whether two hundred and twelve degrees was the cause of the boiling in the instances observed."

"The proposition that all reasoning is deductive may be proved by a similar argument using another intuitive principle;— no event happens without a cause.

"Every case of induction proper proceeds upon the same grounds and in the same way. It is, therefore, evident that induction is no exception to the rule that *inference is always from generals to particulars, and not from particulars to generals.*

"Reasoning by analogy proceeds in the same way; the difference is only in the character of the first premise, which is, that similar causes *are likely* to produce similar effects, or that things that agree in certain attributes or relations are likely to agree in certain other attributes or relations."

It is evident that, in order to reason, the mind must have some general ideas and judgments that are conceived intuitively, and not formed by mere addition or generalization; for nothing is gained by making a class of individuals or particulars, and then drawing one or more out again.

Some of the earliest are: Every body is in space. No event happens without a cause. Like material causes produce like effects.

"It is the province of psychology to explain under what circumstances these primary ideas are given by the senses, the consciousness and the reason; but logic assumes their existence as the indispensable basis of inference, and its appropriate office is to explain in what way we infer one judgment from another.

"*The process of reasoning, when completed, is found to be simply this: Something is predicated, that is, affirmed or denied of a class; an individual is affirmed to belong to this class, and then, of course the same thing can be affirmed or denied of that individual.*"

When the student perceives that the foundation of homœopathy is solid *concrete,* composed of the broken rock of hard facts, united by the *cement* of a great natural principle, he has grasped one important phase of the subject. But when he raises his eyes to the superstructure and sees that it is joined to the foundation, and held together in all its parts by *a framework of logic,* he has gained possession of the key that not only admits him to the edifice, but unlocks the door of every room in it.

Jevons truly says:—"It is true that we cannot use our eyes or ears without getting some kind of knowledge, and the brute animals can do the same. *But what gives power is the deeper knowledge called Science.* People may see, and hear, and feel all their lives without really learning the nature of the things they see. But reason is the mind's eye and enables us to see why things are, and when and how events may be made to happen or not to happen. The logician endeavors to learn exactly what this reason is which makes the power of men. We all must reason well or ill, but logic is the science of reasoning and enables us to distinguish between the good reasoning that leads to the truth, and to bad reasoning which every day betrays people into error and misfortune."

Hence the value and need to the physician of the study of inductive logic as a distinct science.

Analysis of the *Organon* of Hahnemann, as well as of the history of homœopathy and the life of its founder, shows clearly that homœopathy is a product of inductive logic applied to the subject of medicine. It is, in fact, the first as well as one of the most brilliant examples of the application of the inductive method to the solution of one of the greatest problems of humanity; namely, the treatment and cure of disease.

Its basic principle, the law of similars, dimly perceived and tentatively stated in various forms or referred to as a possible therapeutic law by Hippocrates, Nicander, Xenocrates, of the Greek schools; Varro, Quintus Serenus, Celsus and Galen of the Roman schools; Basil Valentine, a Benedictine Monk of Erfurt, 1410; Paracelsus, in the sixteenth century and others, was conceived by Hahnemann to be the general law of medical action.

With this conception as a starting point Hahnemann began to investigate. He reasoned that if there was any truth in the proposition that "diseases are cured by medicines that have the power to excite a *similar affection*," the only way to determine it scientifically would be to give a medicine to *a healthy person* and observe the effects, since a healthy person would be the only kind of a person in whom *an affection similar to disease* could be excited.

This would give a scientific basis, and indeed the only possible basis, for a comparison between the symptoms of drugs and the symptoms of disease.

Accordingly, as every homœopathist knows, he began to experiment with "good cinchona bark" upon himself, that drug having been suggested to him while he was translating Cullen's work on materia medica, where it was highly recommended as a cure for intermittent fever. Finding his theory strikingly confirmed by repeated experiments, he began to search medical literature for records of poisonings and accidental cures. Collecting these as a basis for further experiment and corroboration, he enlisted the aid of a few students and physicians and continued his experiments upon the healthy, carefully recording all the phenomena elicited and verifying them in the sick as he had opportunity.

After several years of this work he had a collection of reliable drug phenomena so large and comprehensive that he felt he could complete the induction and independently and authoritatively formulate the general principle which he had so long been working to establish.

This is Hahnemann's chief contribution to science. He was the first to make a comprehensive induction of medical facts, deduce therefrom the general law of therapeutic medication and establish healing by medication upon a sound basis.

Thus we see that although Hahnemann's primary conception was one of those rare flashes of insight or intuition vouchsafed only to transcendent genius, it was subsequently developed by logical reasoning and confirmed by a series of elaborate experiments extending over a period of many years, before it was published to the world.

When the relation of these facts to the practice of homœopathy is perceived it is evident that in logic the homœopathic physician has, or may have, the means not only of conducting his daily work with ease and facility, but of solving his most difficult and important problems; *for the logical process by which homœopathy was worked out and built up is applicable in every concrete case a homœopathic physician is called upon to treat.* The principles are the same with each case. The examination of a patient or a prover; the analysis of the mass of symptoms derived from such an examination; the classification of symptoms for any purpose; the selection of the remedy and the diagnosis of the disease are all properly conducted under the rules and by the methods of applied logic.

As applied in the examination of a patient, the principles of inductive logic lead the examiner first to gather all the facts of a case and to complete each symptom by careful inquiry into its origin, its exciting or occasioning cause or causes; its history and duration; its relations to other symptoms; and its modalities or modifying circumstances and conditions.

Logic then, by the processes of analysis, synthesis, comparison and generalization makes it possible to determine the relative value and importance, from the prescriber's standpoint, of every symptom. It thus furnishes the means of discovering "characteristic symptoms," which are of such importance in the study of the case.

"**Characteristic Symptoms.**"—Characteristic symptoms are *general symptoms,* or generalizations, inferred or deduced from particular symptoms by the logical process of generalizing.

By generalizing we learn what is true of many different things; that in which they agree or have in common.

Considering the symptoms of Pulsatilla, for example, we find that they agree in all being worse in a warm room or better in the open air. "Aggravation in a warm room" therefore is a "keynote," a "characteristic," or a "general" of Pulsatilla. These terms are used to describe or epitomize those peculiar features which characterize the patient as an individual; facts that are *true of the case as a whole;* or of a number of the particular symptoms of the case, considered as a group. In other words "characteristics" are the individualizing factors of a case or remedy. They are the points which enable us to differentiate between similar cases and remedies. After deducing the general features of a given case or remedy and logically grouping them, thus determining its individuality, we are in a position to compare it with other similar, related remedies or cases for classification, selection of the curative remedy, or any other purpose.

Pathological Unity of Symptoms.—The inductive method brings into view *the pathological unity of the symptoms* of which diseases consist, enabling us to identify and name the various forms they take.

Speaking generally, the internal, invisible, abnormal state of the organism which we call disease, is made manifest externally by perceptible symptoms. If it were necessary only to consider each symptom separately, without regard to the individuality of the general abnormal condition which they represent, we might place the symptoms of disease in numerical order, like words in a dictionary, and select the similar medicine by a mere mechanical comparison of symptom with symptom. But in this case we should be working only with particulars, none of which, taken singly, discloses the individuality of either the disease or the remedy. (Hempel.)

Every disease is the result of the action upon the living organism of some definite, specific, individual agent or influence from without, and the phenomena of its action as a whole take on individualizing general characteristics. By these we identify, name and classify diseases as well as medicines. The names, pneumonia, diphtheria, measles, smallpox, typhoid fever, and many others, represent pathological forms which are, in their characteristic general features, constant in all ages and countries. They owe their existence to causes which are constant, although particular symptoms and the conditions of their manifestations may vary in individual cases and at different periods. We must not lose sight of this essential fact:—that pathological symptoms in definite diseases derive their meaning and relative value from their connection with a definite, general pathological condition or state, exactly as pathogenetic symptoms derive their meaning and value from an individual definite drug, the action of which upon the vital substance they manifest and express.

In order to recognize these pathogenetic and pathological forms, therefore, we resort to the processes of inductive logic; namely, observation and collection of particular facts or phenomena, from the consideration of which we arrive at a conception of the nature and individual character of the groups by the process of generalization.

Totality of the Symptoms.—Logic facilitates the comprehension of the related totality or picture of the symptoms of the case as a whole. From all the parts, logic constructs the whole. It reveals the case; in other words, by generalizing it assigns each detail to its proper place and gives concrete form to the case so that it may be grasped by the mind in its entirety.

The true "totality" is more than the mere numerical totality or whole number of the symptoms. It may even exclude some of the particular symptoms if they cannot, at the time, be logically related to the case. Such symptoms are called "accidental symptoms," and are not allowed to influence the choice of the remedy. The "totality" is that concrete form which the symptoms take when they are logically related to each other and stand forth as an individuality, recognizable by anyone who is familiar with the symptomatic forms and lineaments of drugs and diseases.

The basis of homœopathic prescription is the totality of the symptoms of the patient, *as viewed and interpreted from the standpoint of the prescriber.* A successful prescription cannot be made from the standpoint of the diagnostician, the surgeon nor the pathologist, as such, because of the differing interpretation and classification of symptoms. *A prescription can only be made upon those symptoms which have their counterpart or similar in the materia medica.*

A surgical or a diagnostic symptom may perhaps be elaborated or interpreted into the terms of materia medica, but unless this can be done it is of no value to the prescriber. It is entirely a matter of interpretation and classification. Given all the ascertainable facts in a case (the numerical totality), the representative of each department in medicine selects, defines and interprets those facts which are of use to him in accordance with the demands of his own department; whether there be several individuals acting or only one individual acting in several capacities.

Individualization.—The practical work of the prescriber in constructing the totality or "case" and selecting the remedy is governed throughout by the logical principle of individualization. It applies equally in the three departments of his work.

1. The examination of the patient. This must be conducted in such a manner as to bring out all the facts of the case. Each symptom, as far as possible, must be rendered complete in the three elements of locality, sensation, and modality, or conditions of existence.

2. The examination of the symptom-record of the patient, or the "study of the case." This must be made in such a manner as to determine what symptoms represent that which is curable by medication, under the law of similars; in other words, to determine, in each particular case, what symptoms have a counterpart in the materia medica.

3. The examination of the materia medica, by means of

indexes, repertories, etc., for the purpose of discovering that remedy which, in its symptomatology, is most similar to the symptoms of the individual patient, at a particular time.

To individualize is to confer particular characteristics upon, distinguish. To select or mark as individual; note the peculiar properties of; particularize; characterize.

"Individualization" has been the burden of the message of every great teacher since Hahnemann. But too often they have failed or omitted to state the principles upon which the process of individualization is based. They have reported cases illustrating their own personal method of selecting the curative remedy, by which they have attained marvelous results; but they have not shown us fully the inner workings of their minds. They have formulated certain rules, but few or none of these rules are of general application. We are like the man from Missouri; we "want to be shown." We want to know the "why" as well as the "how." We want principles as well as rules.

It was not because they were unwilling, nor that they did not try to reveal the secret of their great skill and power as prescribers. To some of their personal students, with whom they were in peculiar sympathy, they at least partly succeeded in imparting their secret. It is probable, however, that most of these fortunate students received more by unconscious absorption or by intuition than they did by direct verbal instruction. It is doubtful if they themselves always recognized and identified the mental process by which they did their work. If they did, they neglected to *name it*.

Simple, even trivial as it seems, the omission to *name* a thing or a process, once it is known and used, leads to almost endless trouble and confusion. In its outworking it is sometimes tragical. "A name," quaintly says Hobbes, "is a word taken at pleasure to serve for a small mark which may raise in our mind a thought like to some thought we had before, and which being pronounced to others, may be to them a sign of what thought the speaker had before in his mind." Names then are contrivances for economizing language: But this is not their sole function. It is by their means that we are enabled to assert general propositions; to affirm or deny any predicate of an indefinite number of things at once. (Mill.)

Had our teachers of materia medica and therapeutics told us, simply, that they were using the logical faculty in their work, the faculty by which we *reason* upon facts and propositions; and that the principles which governed them were the principles of *Applied Logic,* we should have been directed at once to the science which, above all others, tends to elucidate the problems that meet us at every step in our medical career and saved us much groping in dark places.

In order to perform successfully the various processes that make up the work of the homœopathic prescriber, he must use his reason in a scientific manner, that is logically; for logic is the Science of Reasoning.

These seem like truisms until we watch the work of the ordinary prescriber and find that instead of doing this, he is merely using *his memory* of a few facts and a few inadequate or erroneous rules which he has picked up. This is empiricism, not science. In an art which has to do with the saving of human life, it is a crime.

Science is the application of *principles* to art and life. Principles are deduced from facts by the exercise of reason. Reasoning is conducted according to fixed laws, which it is our business to learn and apply. To learn how to reason scientifically upon the facts of his department is as essential for the homœopathic physician as it is for any other scientific man.

Great medical artists, men like Hahnemann, Boenninghausen, Hering, Lippe, Dunham, Wells, Guernsey, Fincke, had logical minds, and used the methods and processes of applied logic, perhaps without realizing that they were doing so. They were great by natural endowment as well as by attainment. The special value of their work for us in this connection lies, not in the great number of characteristics and particular indications for treatment which they discovered and published; nor in their valuable manuals and repertories; but in the fact that they possessed and used certain general principles, by the application of which, when they are made known, we, as well as they, may individualize each case and remedy and discover its characteristics for ourselves.

The Art of Generalizing.—Analysis, comparison, classification, and generalization are the logical processes by means of which the homœopathic artist accomplishes his purpose, which is the individualization of his case and the selection of the similar remedy therefor.

Of these processes, generalization, being the synthesis or summing up of the results of the preceding work, is perhaps the most important. Certainly it is the one which is least understood and most neglected in ordinary practice; and yet without it, it is impossible to do good work.

The greater includes the less. Generals are more important than particulars in constructing a case and as a basis for prescribing. The generals, which include and are derived from the particulars, constitute the only reliable basis of a curative prescription. Generalizing, therefore, is one of the most important functions performed by the homœopathic prescriber in selecting the curative medicine.

Mill, in his Treatise on Logic, says: "A general truth is but an aggregate of particular truths; a comprehensive expression by which an indefinite number of individual facts are affirmed or denied at once." A generalization is the process of obtaining a general conception, rule or law, from a consideration of particular facts or phenomena. A generalization is not possible until the mind has grasped and assimilated all the particulars which enter into its formation. Then they take on form and individuality and are seen as a whole. The mind recognizes and perhaps names the identity, or describes its characteristics in comprehensive phrase. Details enter into minor generalizations, and minor generalizations into major, until one all-inclusive concept or principle is seen and stated. Such is *Similia Similibus Curantur,* one of the most far-reaching generalizations ever made by the mind of man. Its scope no man has ever yet compassed. We have a fair comprehension of its application in healing the sick by the use of medicine, but of its application in the realm of ethics, for example, to which it obviously stands related, we have only begun to have an inkling.

The value of a generalization depends primarily upon the data from which it is drawn. We have seen that these must be accurate and complete. The mistake is constantly being made of attempting to generalize from insufficient, incorrect or hastily gathered data. This is as true of the homœopathic doctor who rushes into the sick room, asks a few hurried questions, looks at the nurse's chart and makes a "snap-shot prescription" as it is of the pathologist who jumps to the conclusion that microbes are the ultimate cause of disease because he has failed to see with his microscope what lies in the surrounding field.

General Symptoms.—*The patient sometimes correctly generalizes parts of his own case.* This he may do quite unconsciously, as when he refers certain symptoms or conditions of symptoms to his inner consciousness by saying, "I feel" thus and so; "*I am* worse in rainy weather;" "*I am* sad, or depressed, or easily angered" as the case may be.

Nearly all mental symptoms are generals because mental states can only be expressed in general terms.

Psychologically an emotion or a passion such as anger, grief or jealousy, *is a complex state of consciousness* in which one or more forms of excited sensibility are expanded, made sensuous and strengthened by admixture of various peripheral or organic sensations that are aroused by some primary feeling. The process by which we become aware of the resulting concrete emotion and give it a name, is essentially *a generalization, subconsciously performed.* For this reason mental symptoms, when they appear in the record of a case, are always of the highest rank as material for the final generalization and completion of the totality upon which the prescription is based.

The most intimate and interior things; the things that lie nearest to the heart of man; the things that touch and express the centers of life, are among the generals.

Statements or observations that reflect a man's state of mind, his moods, his passions, his fears, his desires and aversions, are all generals because they express the man himself and not merely some part or organ. "The mind is the man."

Symptoms that express the subconscious or involuntary actions of the mind, such as the manner of sleeping, peculiar or unusual positions assumed during sleep or disease, character of dreams or delirium, are generals.

"Modalities, or conditions of aggravation and amelioration applying to the case as a whole, or the patient himself, are **generals of high rank.**" (Kent.)

Particular symptoms, or those which express the suffering of some part, organ, or function of the body have a two-fold use. They are the data from which the general symptoms are drawn; and they are sometimes the differentiating factors between two or more remedies arrived at by exclusion in the comparison of general symptoms.

"Particulars that are included in generals may be left out. Nothing in particulars can contradict or contra-indicate strongly marked generals, though they may appear to do so. 'Aggravation from heat' will exclude Arsenic from any case." (Kent.) (Except a certain form of headache, which is relieved by cold applications.)

Negative General Symptoms.—Absence of certain striking or customary features of a disease may be a general symptom of a case.

Fever without thirst, coldness with aversion to being covered, hunger without appetite, exanthematous diseases without appearance of the eruption, are examples of these negative generals. Every one of the illustrative symptoms given has been determined by the logical process of generalization.

The materia medica is full of such generalizations. There, the work has already been completed and recorded. It is in the clinical cases, at the bedside, or in the office, that the physician must do his own generalizing. Hence the necessity for familiarizing himself with logic and the inductive method in Science.

Grading and Grouping.—Upon correct generalizing depends all successful work as a homœopathic prescriber. Mere mechanical comparison of one particular symptom with another is but little better than "pathological prescribing." The simillimum will but rarely be found by either method. As well might a general expect to win a battle by trying to direct each individual soldier in his army against each individual soldier in the enemies' army. He must grade and group his men into companies, his companies into regiments, his regiments into brigades and the whole into a great army, and direct its movements as a whole. The individual soldier is the unit of strength, but the units must be massed and graded and drilled according to scientific principles until they act as one man. This gives what the French significantly call *"esprit de corps."* The army of individuals then comes to have an individuality as an army, one spirit and purpose permeating the whole. In like manner must the symptoms of a proving, or of a case of sickness, be graded and grouped and studied, until the individuality of the remedy or the case appears distinct and clear before the mind.

The study of materia medica and the study of disease are conducted in a similar manner, for they are counterparts. The materia medica is a *fac simile* of the sickness of humanity in all its phases and features.

Memorizing Symptoms.—The attempt to obtain a practical grasp or working knowledge of the materia medica, or even of a single remedy by merely *memorizing details* or single symptoms will always fail. The provings must be so studied as to impress upon the mind and memory an image, or concept of the *individuality of the drug as a whole*, so that it may be recognized as we recognize any other individual or person. The memorizing of single symptoms, peculiar in themselves, has its place and value, but it is secondary in the larger scheme under discussion.

When a miscellaneous collection of data is submitted to the logically trained mind for comprehension, it immediately begins to compare phenomena according to some comprehensive plan, in order that it may discover general characteristics, if possible, which may again be grouped in such a manner as to develop form and individuality in the whole. This is generalizing, and is the method employed in the construction of materia medica from the provings. In this way "keynotes" or "characteristic symptoms" are discovered. A "keynote" may be defined as a concise statement of a single characteristic feature of a drug deduced by a critical consideration of its symptoms as recorded in a proving. In other words it is a minor generalization based upon a study of particulars. It is not usually a single symptom as stated or observed by a prover in describing his sensations, for that which is characteristic in any large way of a drug is rarely shown in a single symptom. Thus the statement that the Pulsatilla case is "worse in a close or warm room" is a generalization drawn from the observation of particular symptoms in numerous cases, both in provings and clinically. The same is true of nearly every condition of aggravation and amelioration contained in Boenninghausen's Repertory, the greatest masterpiece of analysis comparison and generalization in our literature. Experience has shown that most of these "conditions" or modalities of Boenninghausen are *general in their relations.* The attempt to limit the application of the modality to the particular symptoms with which they were first observed has not led to success in prescribing. Boenninghausen did his work well, and he followed strictly the inductive method. Of these modalities he wrote: "All of these indications are so trustworthy, and have been verified by such manifold experiences, that hardly any others can equal them in rank—to say nothing of surpassing them. But the most valuable fact respecting them is this: That this characteristic is not confined to one or another symptom, *but like a red thread it runs through all the morbid symptoms of a given remedy, which are associated with any kind of pain whatever,* or even with a sensation of discomfort, and hence it is available for both internal and external symptoms of the most varied character." In other words, they are general characteristics deduced by a critical study of particulars and verified in practice.

Dramatizing the Materia Medica.—"Personification" of remedies by artistic character delineation is an interesting form of materia medica study for those who have a highly developed imagination.

This attempts to bring before the mind's eye, the imagination, a picture of the drug in human form, as an individual, whose features we may recognize as we do those of a friend whom we meet on the street. The artist draws the symptom portrait of a man, or a woman, as the case may be. He introduces us to a personality. Taking the material furnished by the prover and following anatomical and physiological lines, he delineates a human figure, first in bold and sweeping outlines, then in finer and more characteristic touches which give individuality. Even the mental traits and peculiarities are there. True, a sick man is portrayed, but none the less does he possess the traits of humanity. We do not love our friends the less when they are sick. They may even possess additional elements of interest for us because they are sick. And so these ghostly forms which the materia medica wizard conjures up out of the "vasty deep" are friends of ours and allies; inhabitants of a "spirit-world" from whence they are ever ready to appear at our behest. Our knowledge of the law of cure and of potentiation gives us control over such spirits, and we may say, with the disciples of old, "even the devils are subject to us,"—for substances like Crotalus or Lachesis, deadly serpent poisons, which, in their crude state, possess properties simply devilish in their terrible malignity, by dilution and potentiation become beneficent healing remedies full of blessing to suffering mankind.

Generalizing for Repertory Work.—In using repertories, notably "Boenninghausen," which all Hahnemannian prescribers use, we constantly generalize. We bring together and correlate the partial, disconnected statements of the patient into complete and rounded wholes which may, perhaps, be characterized by a single word corresponding to a rubric in the repertory. Take, for example, the word "maliciousness," classified by Boenninghausen under the general heading "mind." At first thought that would seem to be a particular symptom; but a little reflection will show it to be a generalization, drawn from a number of observations. Rarely will a patient state, or even admit on being directly questioned, that he is maliciously disposed. If it is a fact it will be deduced by the discerning physician from a number of facts, learned directly by the inductive process. The same is true of a great number of mental states. We become aware of them in the course of our careful observation and study of the case, by piecing together detached bits of evidence.

Generalizing the mental states is the most difficult of all and requires the exercise of the highest powers of the physician. In difficult cases of nervous and mental disease the physician must be a trained psychologist and a logician, as well as a most alert and accurate observer.

Reviewing and summarizing the ground thus far covered we find that the inductive method in science is cumulative and evolutionary. It eliminates every element of speculation and deals only with established facts. It takes nothing for granted when data are concerned. It ignores no fact, no matter how trifling it may seem. It confines its operations strictly within the limits of the subject directly in hand. Its deductions are always direct, never indirect. It never makes an inference or deduction from a process of reasoning, or from theoretical grounds, but always from carefully observed facts. A generalization made according to the principles of Inductive Logic stands in direct and logical relation with the data from which it is drawn and includes them in their essential features. It is arrived at through a series of steps or degrees, in which each conclusion rests firmly upon the preceding steps.

The principles which govern the art of generalization may be summarized as follows:

1. The mind must be freed from the bias of pre-conceived opinions and theories.

2. The subject must be clearly defined, or restricted within definite limits.

3. The phenomena must be determined by actual observation or experimentation, with a single end in view; viz., the truth.

4. All the phenomena must be gathered, if possible. No fact must be omitted, however trifling it may seem.

5. No phenomena are to be admitted to the induction of a study but those elicited by its own process in its own province.

6. The facts must be clearly expressed and recorded with exactness and precision.

7. The phenomena must be expressed and recorded in terms of simple fact, free from speculation about their causes.

8. The facts having been ascertained and clearly stated, they are to be arranged in their natural relation to each other and to the subject of the inquiry by comparison and generalization.

9. Generalization proceeds by bringing together similar and related phenomena into groups, considering these in their relation to each other and to other groups, deducing their general characteristics and stating them in simple, comprehensive form.

10. Particulars appropriately grouped lead to minor generalizations, which in turn lead to greater generalizations, but always as required by Lord Bacon's formula, "ascending continually and by degrees." "The most rigorous conditions of gradual and successive generalizations must be adopted."

11. Nothing should be deduced from the facts of observation except what they inevitably include.

12. At every stage of the investigation, the analysis of the phenomena must be carried to its utmost limits before the process of synthesis is begun.

The Law of Causation.—The science of logic has an important relation to medicine in the matter of assigning the causes of disease, upon which, as far as possible, treatment is based. If treatment is to be governed to any extent by the idea of removing or counteracting the effects of the cause of the disease, it follows that success will depend upon correct conclusions as to what constitutes the cause or causes.

Many, if not most, of the mistakes and failures in medical treatment are due to the failure to comprehend and correctly apply the principle of logic known as the *Law of Causation.*

Everyone is quite ready to agree that "every effect must have a cause." But investigation shows that very few seem to know, or, if they know, make use of their knowledge of the fact, that *every effect has a number of causes,* all of which must be taken into consideration if correct conclusions are to be formed.

Mill (System of Logic) says:

"The theory of *Induction* is based upon the notion of *Cause*. The truth that every fact which has a beginning has a cause is co-extensive with human experience. The recognition of this truth and its formation into a law, from which other laws are derived, is a generalization from the observed facts of nature, upon which all true science is based."

"The phenomena of nature exist in two distinct relations to one another; that of *simultaneity,* and that of *succession*. Every phenomenon is related, in a uniform manner, to some phenomena which co-exist with it, and to some that have preceded and will follow it."

"Of all truths relating to phenomena the most valuable are those which relate to the order of their succession. On a knowledge of these is founded every reasonable anticipation of future facts, and whatever power we possess of influencing those facts to our advantage. From the same knowledge do we derive our power to make the most effective use of past and present facts."

"When we speak of the cause of any phenomena, we do not mean a cause which is not itself a phenomenon. It is not necessary (in practice) to invade the realm of metaphysics and seek for the ultimate cause of anything. Of the essences and inherent constitution of things we can know nothing. The only notion of a cause which the theory of induction requires is such a notion as can be gained by experience, in the correct observation and interpretation of facts. But much depends upon how we observe facts. The trustworthiness of facts often depends upon the accuracy and freedom from prejudice of the observer. Inasmuch as we do not reason from facts, but from *our conception of the facts,* it follows that the reliability of our conclusions depends not only upon correct observation and correct reasoning, but upon the truthfulness of our conceptions of facts."

(Jevons says: "Science is in the mind and not in things.")

"The Law of Causation, which is the main pillar of inductive science, is but the recognition of the familiar truth that between the phenomena which exist at any instant and the phenomena which exist at the succeeding instant, there is an invariable order of succession. To certain facts, certain facts always do, and, as we believe, will continue to succeed. The invariable antecedent is termed the cause; the invariable consequent, the effect."

"The universality of the law of causation consists in this, that every consequent is connected in this manner with some particular antecedent, or set of antecedents. Let the fact be what it may, if it has begun to exist, it was preceded by some fact or facts, with which it is invariably connected. For every event there exists some combination of objects or events, some given concurrence of circumstances, positive or negative, the occurrence of which is always followed by that phenomenon. We may not have found out what the concurrence of circumstances may be; but we never doubt that there is such a one, and that it never occurs without having the phenomenon in question as its effect on consequence."

"It is seldom, if ever, between a consequent and a single antecedent that this invariable sequence subsists. It is usually between the consequent and the sum of several antecedents; the concurrence of all of them being requisite to produce, that is, to be certain of being followed by, the consequent."

"In such cases it is very common to single out one only of

the antecedents under the domination of Cause, calling the others merely Conditions: Thus, if a person eats of a particular dish, and dies in consequence, that is, would not have died if he had not eaten of it, people would be apt to say that eating of that dish was the cause of his death. There need not, however, be any invariable connection between eating of the dish and death; but there certainly is, among the circumstances which took place, some combination or other on which death is invariably consequent; as, for instance, the act of eating of the dish, combined with a particular bodily constitution, a particular state of present health, and perhaps even a certain state of the atmosphere; the whole of which circumstances perhaps constituted in this particular case the *conditions* of the phenomenon, or in other words, the set of antecedents which determined it, and but for which it would not have happened."

"*The real cause is the whole of these antecedents, and we have no right, philosophically speaking, to give the name of the cause to one of them, exclusively of the others.*"

The most common, and in its outworkings the most pernicious medical error, is to assume that a disease or a morbid condition had a *single* cause, and to direct all efforts and agencies against that.

This error is responsible for such tragic failures as have resulted from the attempts to treat or eradicate cholera, tuberculosis and diphtheria on the assumption, at least virtually, that bacilli were the sole cause of these diseases.

The mortality in the last great cholera epidemic under antibacillar treatment was the greatest in history. Human tuberculosis under the same *regime* continues its ravages unabated, while millions of dollars worth of cattle have been uselessly destroyed in the attempt to stamp out bovine tuberculosis.

In 1915, after about fifteen years of experience, the Department of Health of New York City, in its official Weekly Bulletin, December 18, 1915, announced the total failure of diphtheria-antitoxin and all other measures of treatment based upon the bacilli hypothesis to reduce or control the prevalence of diphtheria.

Reporting a conference held at the Department of Health, it said:—

"Thus it was generally agreed that the prevalence of diphtheria was as great, or even greater now as it was years ago, although, of course, (Sic) the mortality from that disease has been very greatly reduced. In other words, although the administrative efforts of the health authorities—that is, the provision of facilities for early diagnosis and the introduction in the number of the Antitoxin treatment has produced a striking reduction in the number of deaths, they have been wholly without influence on the number of cases occurring."

The oriental expedient of trying to "save face" by emphasizing reduced mortality is as shallow as the former claims of ability to reduce and control the prevalency of the disease; for it can easily be shown that the reduced mortality is due more to other causes, some of them purely natural, than measures based upon the bacillar hypothesis.

The ridiculous "Swat the Fly" campaigns, enthusiastically conducted in various parts of the country in recent times, afford another example of the prevailing ignorance of the law of causation. Of what use is it to "swat the fly" while no attention is given to the uncovered garbage pails, the reeking manure heaps and privy-vaults and the numerous other filth centers which are his breeding places?

Ignorance or misapprehension of the Law of Causation is the strongest and most serious indictment that has been brought against the advocates of bacteriology as a foundation for therapeutics. Brilliant and successful as have been the attainments of bacteriologists in creating a new science of sanitary engineering, they have failed, and must continue to fail, to establish bacteriology as the basis of a true therapeutics. The fatal tendency in this department of medical research to focus attention and effort upon *one* cause to the exclusion of all others inevitably leads into error and failure.

In cholera, for example, admitting the existence and presence of the bacilli as one causative factor, we still have to reckon with sanitary, atmospheric and telluric conditions; with economic and social conditions and habits of life; with means and modes of transportation and intercommunication between individuals and communities; with individual physical, mental and emotional states, etc., all of which are essential factors, in some combination, in determining and modifying the susceptibility of individuals to the bacilli; for without some combination of these factors the bacilli are impotent and the disease would never occur. Each of these factors is a cause at least equal in rank with the bacilli, and any successful method of treatment must be able to meet all the conditions arising from any existing combination of the causes.

This may seem like an impossible requirement, but experience proves that homœopathy, with a mortality record in cholera as low as four per cent and less, against a record as high as seventy per cent under other forms of treatment, is able to meet it. The secret of this success is that homœopathy does not direct its efforts primarily or solely to the destruction of the *proximate physical cause* of the disease (the micro-organism), but against *the disease itself;* that is, *the morbid vital process as manifested by the symptoms,* using symptomatically similar medicines capable of causing a *counter action* of the organism *similar* in nature to that of the pathogenic agent, neutralizing its effects and thus restoring systemic balance, or health.

"From nothing, from a mere negation, no consequence can proceed. All effects are connected, by the law of causation, with some set of *positive* conditions; negative ones, it is true, being almost always required in addition. In other words, every fact or phenomenon which has a beginning, invariably arises when some certain combination of positive facts exists, provided certain other positive facts do not exist." (Mill.)

Thus diphtheria may be prevalent in a community, and the specific micro-organisms (Klebs-Loeffler bacilli) of that disease be present in the throats of many healthy individuals; but if those individuals have a high or sufficient resistance to the action of the bacilli, and are not therefore susceptible to infection, they destroy the bacilli and escape the disease. The necessary combination of positive facts and conditions does not exist for them.

The power of the bacilli or other infectious agents is always relative and conditional, never absolute, as many are led to believe. The bacilli, therefore, are not the sole cause of the disease, but only one possible factor in a group or combination of causes or conditions, all of which must exist and act together before the disease can follow.

CHAPTER XVII

The Development of Hahnemannian Philosophy in the Sixth Edition of "The Organon"

When it was announced that the long-awaited Sixth Edition of Hahnemann's "Organon" was at last available and about to be published, there was great curiosity on the part of his present-day followers to see what changes, additions or developments were embodied in it.

What subjects had most interested and occupied the mind of the Old Master during the last years of his long life? What subjects did he regard as the most important and as most needing further elucidation? Had he changed his mind in regard to any of the fundamental principles of his philosophy? Had he formed any new theories? Had he changed his method of applying the principles which he had laid down in former editions?

Speculation on these questions was rife. There were some, like the writer, who believed that few changes would be found in the practical rules and methods which had stood the test of more than a century of experience and proved their permanent value in the cure of innumerable cases of disease. They expected that the changes would consist of a further development and elucidation of those theories and concepts which constituted the latest former additions to his system—abstruse subjects which did not appear or were only lightly touched upon in the early editions; subjects, for example, like those of vitality, dynamism and potentiation, which were the last to be developed and introduced into the "Organon."

This conjecture turned out to be correct, and it is well for the medical world that it did. Never was there greater need than now that the medical profession should be reminded, as by a voice from the celestial world, that there is something more vital and more important for them and for suffering humanity than matter and materialism; than germs and germicides; than serums and vaccines; than mechanics and mechanisms; than pathological processes and products.

That "Something" is a fuller knowledge and realization of the spiritual nature of life or mind in organism; of life or mind as a spiritual, entitative power or principle manifesting itself in and through the physical organisms of which it is the architect and builder as-well as the tenant.

Whatever tends to throw light upon the connection between mind and body; whatever enlarges or clarifies our conceptions of what Life is and how it builds its house, or performs its functions; whatever enlarges our knowledge of the relations between the various organs and systems of organs of the physical body; whatever tends to show how the living organism acts and reacts under the influence of external or internal agencies—mental, psychical or physical; that is important, and important in the highest degree, because the medical profession as a whole has largely neglected or ignored these phases of the subject and has regarded man merely as a mechanism actuated solely by physical forces—and treated him accordingly. From this misconception arise the most glaring errors, the most flagrant abuses and the most tragical results in the medical and surgical treatment of today.

Hahnemann, in his later life, with marvelous insight and striking prescience, fixed his attention principally upon the spiritual and dynamical aspects of the subject of medicine. Hence we find that the changes, additions and developments in the Sixth Edition of "The Organon" deal principally with these subjects. These remained longest in his mind. To them he gave his deepest and most mature thought. Evidently he regarded the results of his thought as sufficiently important to justify a new, and, as he termed it "most likely the last" edition of his immortal masterpiece, "THE ORGANON."

Dynamism, The Vital Force, Potentiation and the Infinitesimal Dose: Around these three subjects have centered the hottest controversies and most mordant criticisms in the history of homœopathy; and these are the newly treated subjects in the Sixth Edition of "The Organon." For more than a century the battle between the "dynamists" and the "materialists" has been fought—the "dynamists" always in the minority, but unconquer-

THE DEVELOPMENT OF HAHNEMANNIAN PHILOSOPHY 273

able. Their heads are "bloody but unbowed." The "long, thin line" is unbroken. Their trenches are deep and well protected. Their supplies of ammunition are constantly being replenished and their weapons improved by the latest findings and conclusions of modern science, the whole trend of which is toward the confirmation of the dynamical conclusions arrived at by Hahnemann.

The invention of the telegraph, telephone, electric dynamo, X-ray machine, phonograph, telegraphone, "radio," the discovery of radium, etc.; the advances made in the study and utilization of electronic and ionic machines, and of colloids and solutions in general—The New Dynamism—these have all been brought about in physical science through the application of the identical dynamical principles which Hahnemann was among the first to recognize in their general application, and the first to apply in modern medicine and therapeutics.

To Hahnemann belongs the honor of having been the first physician to connect biology and psychology with physics in a practical system of medicinal therapeutics, and to give an impulse to studies in biodynamics which has gained momentum continuously ever since.

When Hahnemann, after formulating his principal concepts of Life or Mind in its relation to the physical organism, began to experiment with the action of drugs upon healthy human subjects, observing the subjective as well as the objective phenomena, he opened up a new field of research and laid the foundation for a true science and art of medicine and psychology. From that time forward, and for the first time, man could be studied and treated scientifically as an individual, in all his personal and peculiar actions and reactions.

The philosophy of Hahnemann is based upon and includes not only the physiological and pathological actions and reactions of man as a physical organism, but of man as a spiritual and psychical being; for it includes and utilizes the mental, the subjective and the functional phenomena as they are developed under the influence of hygeopoietic and pathogenetic agencies. In this respect homœopathy differs radically from and is infinitely superior to all other systems of therapeutics; and this is solely because it recognizes Life or Mind as an entity; as the primary, spiritual power or principle which creates and sustains the physical organism and is the primary cause of all its actions and reactions. Its working principle is the universal Law of Reciprocal Action, otherwise known as the law of balance, compensation, rhythm, polarity, vibration, or action and reaction, all of which signify a principle operative alike in the physical, mental and spiritual realms. In its out-working it is essentially the *Law of Love,* for it is always beneficent, always creative, always harmonizing. Hence, the consistent practitioner of homœopathy never uses, and has no need to use, any irritating, weakening, depressing, infecting, intoxicating or injurious agent of any kind in the treatment of the sick, nor to violate the integrity of the body by forcibly introducing medicinal agents by other than the natural orifices and channels.

Homœopathy achieves its ends and accomplishes its purposes by the use of single, simple, pure drugs; refined and deprived of their injurious properties and enhanced in curative power by the pharmacodynamical processes of mechanical comminution, trituration, solution and dilution according to scale; in minimum or infinitesimal doses, administered by the mouth; the remedy having been selected by comparison of the symptoms of the sick with the symptoms of drugs produced by tests in healthy human subjects; under the principle of symptom—similarity, as enunciated in the maxims, "Similia, Similibus Curantur.—Simplex, Simile, Minimum."

This is homœopathy in a nutshell. It is a shell which some find hard to crack, but when cracked it is found to be packed full of sweet and wholesome meat, *with no worms in it.*

INDEX

A

Advances in general medicine, 55
Age of the patient, 194
Aggravation, the homœopathic, 76, 116, 117, 152
Alcohol, 83
Allen, H. C., 104
Ameke, 31
Amelioration of symptoms, 153
Analysis of the case, 177
Anamnesis, 98
Anaphylaxis, 112, 113
Animate and inanimate bodies and forces, difference between, 10, 14
Anshutz, E. P., 94
Antecedents and consequents, 267
Antidotal treatment, 107, 108, 109
Antidote, high potency as, 120
Antiseptics, 81
Antitoxin and diphtheria, 268
Archimedes, 217
Aristotle, 15, 29
Arrhenius, 212
Art, defined, 123
  homœopathy an, 19
  and Science, 14
Artifices in examination, 176
"Art Instinct," 14
Assimilation, Fincke on, 233, 234
Atoms, 230
Attraction between drug and organism, 239
  sphere of, 63, 64, 65
Automobile, the human, 75

B

Babel, Tower of, 75
Bacilli, natural resistance to, 270
Bacon, Lord, 15, 27, 248, 249
  Hahnemann's debt to, 27, 28
Bacterial diseases, homœopathy in, 270
Bacterial therapeutics a failure, 269, 270

Bacteriology not a true basis for therapeutics, 105
  relation to homœopathy, 92
Barrett, Judge, opinion, 145
Behring, on tuberculosis, 99
Beliefs and convictions, 175
Billings, 54
Biologists and physicists, evasions of, 36, 64, 65
Biological Science, homœopathy a, 56
Biology confirms homœopathy, 55
Blanks, history, 180
Boenninghausen, 85, 108, 178
  Therapeutic Pocketbook, 163-165
  Repertory, 264
Boericke, William, 164
Bolometer, 230
Burby, J. D., chemist, on infinite dilution, 228
Burroughs, John, 167
Butler, Glentworth, 118
"By-products," 118

C

Cabot, R. C., 54
Case, analysis of, 177
Case, construction of the, 13
Case records, 172
Case as a whole, the, 50
Causation, law of, 104, 266-270
Cause, the real, in logic, 268
Causes and conditions, 10
  of disease, 43
  most common, 119
  conditional, 111
Centrosome, 63, 64
Changeable and unchangeable forces in living organisms, 10-14
Characteristic symptoms, generalizations, 254
"Characteristics" and "Keynotes," 156-162
Cholera, 67, 68, 69, 97
Cholera mortality, 268
Classification of symptoms, 172, 173

"Complications," 118, 119
Concepts, fundamental, 16
Conditional, all action is, 71
   causes of disease are, 111
Confidence of the patient, gaining the, 171
Consequents and antecedents, 267
Conservation of energy, law of, 227
Constitution and temperament, 194
Contraries, rule of, 119
Controversial spirit, 54
Cosmic Life, 33
Crile, Geo. W., 82
Curative action, requirements for, 189
Cure, Hahnemann's definition of, 72, 74
   direction and manner of, 132
   distinguished from recovery, 125, 126
   how effected, 128
   individual, 130
   how manifested, 128
   the morphological factor, 130
   and Recovery, 122-134
   relation of, to disease, 127
   requirements of, 130
Cuvier, 89

D

Dake, Sphere of Similia, 42, 43, 44
Davies, Logic of Mathematics, 28
Daybooks of provers, 155
Diagnostic Idea, the, 153
"Dilutions," 212
Diphtheria and antitoxin, 268
Discovery, Hahnemann's greatest, 32
Disease, causes of, 43
   chronic, 87-92
   defined, 38
   Hahnemann's definition, 72, 73, 74
   nature of, 66, 67, 70
   as process and products, 37, 38
Dosage, Hahnemann's, 189, 190
   law of, 208-211
Doses, opposite effects of large, and small, 55, 56, 184
   physiological, 185
   repetition of, 202-205
Dramatizing the materia medica, 263
Drug diseases, 114-121
   and idiosyncrasies, 111-121
   potential, 238, 240
Dunham, Carroll, 18
Dynamical theory, 34, 240, 242
Dynamics, science of, 59
   vital, 39, 40, 41

Dynamism, 272
"Dynamis, the," 32, 58, 59
Dynamo, central nervous system compared to, 61

E

Effect of remedy, how judged, 205-208
Elective affinity, 241
Electrical analogies of life, 61, 62
Electricity, 217
Electrons, 230
Emboli, 102
Emerson, Ralph Waldo, 246
Empiricism, 241
"End Products" of Disease, 128
Endotoxins, problem of, Ewing, 80
Entity, life an, 32, 64
Entozoa, 43
Errors in prescribing, 155-156
Ether, 231, 235, 236
   and energy, 63
Evasions of biologists and physicists, 36, 64, 65
Ewing, Prof. James, 80
Examination of the Patient, 131, 167-182
   physical, 171
   purpose of the homœopathic, 176
Expectant Treatment inadequate, 126
Experience, the test of dosage, 221
Experimental science, homœopathy an, 19

F

Fictitious diseases, 92
Fincke, B., 213, 233
Forces, changeable and unchangeable, 10-14
Forms of disease fixed, 12
Function and organ, 38
Fundamental concepts, 16
Future of homœopathy, 146

G

General medicine, advances in, 55
   symptoms, 260
   Practitioner, 169, 170
Generalizations, characteristic symptoms are, 254
Generalizing, art of, 258-260
   principles of, 265
   for repertory work, 264

"Genius of the remedy," 154
Gonorrhœa, suppression of, 133
Grading and grouping symptoms, 261
Grauvogl, 8, 14, 223
  on law of dosage, 208-211
Guernsey, Henry N., 157

H

Hahnemann, discoverer of cholera germs, 69
  his greatest discovery, 32
  a substantialist, 26
  working principles of, 30
Habit and environment, 194, 199
Hall, A. Wilford, 232
Health, definition of, 60
Health Dept. N. Y. City, conference on antitoxin, 268, 269
Hektoen, Ludwig, 93
Hering, C., 116, 162
High potencies, aggravation from, 114
  powers of, 137
Histories, clinical, 178
History, family, 180
Hobbes, on names, 257
Holmes, Oliver Wendell, 120
Homœopathic law, validity of, 4
Homœopathician, make-up of, 2
Homœopathy, an art, 19
  confirmed by biology, 55
  definition of, 2-4, 16, 17, 18
  an experimental science, 16, 19
  founded in laws of Life and Motion, 31
  perversions of, 20
  qualifications for the practice of, 2-4
  superiority of, 126
  working principles of, 21, 22
Honesty in practice, 145
Hyoscyamus, involuntary proving of, 136-137
Hypodermic needle, 124, 125

I

Ideal, Hahnemann's new, 122
Idealism, 24
Idiosyncrasy and Drug Disease, 111-121
Image of the disease, 153
Imbalance, morphological, 113

"Imitation of Nature," not art, 123, 125
Immunity, true, 86
"Improbability" in science, 222
Indications for the remedy, most important, 170
Indispositions and the Second Best Remedy, 135-146
Individualization, 51, 52
  logical, 256, 257
Individual responsibilities, 7
Inductive Logic defined, 248
  method in Science, 248
  Philosophy of Bacon, 27
Infinite dilution, 228
Inflammations, 82
Infinitesimals, 213, et seq.
Inorganic substances, relation to living organism, 225
Ionization, 66, 212, 228, 229
  J. D. Burby on, 228, 229
Intensity of the disease, 200
Intercurrent remedies, 202
Interpretations of nature, general, 8-14
Itch, 101

J

Jahr, on potencies, 192, 193
Jesus used a placebo, 192, 193
Jevons, 245
Jones, Prof. Samuel A., on posology, 214
"Jourdain Monsieur," 244

K

Kelvin, Lord, 230
"Keynote System," 157
Klebs-Loeffler bacilli, 71, 170
Koch, 67, 70, 98

L

Langley, S. P., 230
Language of materia medica, 165
Large and small doses, opposite effects of, 55, 56
Latency, doctrine of, 99
Law of cure, existence implied, 129
Law, definition of, 17
  test of validity of, 17
Laws of Nature, Grauvogl on, 8-14
"Leading questions," 172
Least action, law of, 213
"Least Plus," law of, 86

Leprosy, 100, 103
Lewes, George Henry, 34
Liebig, 224, 225
Life, definitions of, 35, 36, 60
 electrical analogies of, 61, 62
Life, a substantial entity, 32, 64
 evolution of, 33
 and mind, 273, 274
 and Motion, homœopathy founded on laws of, 31
Light, 230, 231
Limitation of thought, 33
Lippe, Adolph, on prescribing, 158, 161
Lodge, Sir Oliver, 231, 232, 234, 235
Logic, Formal, 246
 in homœopathy, 244
 Inductive, 247
 relation to practice, 253
 relation to teaching, 258
"Lost, getting," 116, 117
Luminiferous Ether, 217

M

McConkey, Thos. G., 92, 103
Marzinowsky, 103
Mass, 235
Master, who is a, 1
Materialism, 23, 33, 87
Materia Medica, dramatizing the, 263
 the homœopathic, 147
 language of, 165
Mathematics, logic of, 66
Matter and Force, 62
Matter, new conceptions of, 218
Mechanical conditions, 73
 treatment, 129
Metastasis, 101
Medicine, state of, in Hahnemann's time, 28
Medicines, modification of, Hahnemannian process, 220
Memorizing symptoms, 262
Memory prescribers, 258
Mensuration, scale of, 218, 242, 243
Mental states, generalizing, 264
Metaphysical thought legitimate, 34
Miasms, chronic, 88, 95
Mill, J. S., 248, 259, 266
Misfits, medical, 58
Mission of the physician, 29
Modification of medicines, Hahnemannian process, 220
Moeller, 103

Moliere, 244
Morphological imbalance, 113
Morphology, the new, 130, 131
Moses, 100
Motion, defined, 32
Musser, J. H., 54
Mystery in Nature, 236

N

Names, 257
Nature, examples of homœopathy in, 124
 general interpretations of, 8-14
Negative general symptoms, 261
Newton, Sir Isaac, 17
 on constitution of matter, 216
Nihilism, therapeutic, 54
Noeggerath, 91
Nosodes, 202
Novum Organum, Bacon, 28
Nutshell, homœopathy in a, 274

O

Object of prescribing, 38, 39
Objective symptoms, 15
Obligations of Homœopathists, 145
Obnoxious remedies, 124
Observing the patient, 181, 182
Occupational diseases, 89, 98
Opposite action of large and small doses, 184
Opposition to truth, 1
Organic control, 61
Organism, development of, 32
Organizations, dangers of, 5
Organon of Hahnemann, an inductive product, 252
Organon, sixth edition, 271
Osler, 53, 103
Ozanam, 223

P

Palliative treatment, 45-47
Parasitical diseases, 95, 99
Parr's Medical Dictionary, 1819, 96
Particular symptoms, 261
Pasteur, 68-70
Pathogenetic action of drugs, 186
Pathological conditions, 194, 195
"Pathological Unity," 254
Pathology, general, 87-121

INDEX

Patient, gaining confidence of, 171
  observing the, 181, 182
Patient's story, the, 172
Personalities, great, 1
Personification of remedies, 263
Perversions of homœopathy, 3
Pfund (of Johns Hopkins), 231
Phenomena, order of succession, 265
Physiological action of drugs, 185, 187
  doses, 44
Placebo, doctrine of, 140
  use of, 117, 143
Posology, homœopathic, 183-211
Potencies, 212
  working range of, 191
  choice of, 191
Potential, theory of the, 237, 238
Potentiation, homœopathic, defined, 212
  Hahnemann's latest views, 272
  mathematical limits of, 228
  in Nature, 226
  origin of, 214-216
  scientific foundation of, 227
Pottenger, F. M., 48
Power and Force, distinction between, 32
Prejudice, freedom from, 174
Prescribing, errors in, 155, 156
  logical standpoint in, 256
  object of, 38, 39
Primary entity, 33
  and Secondary action of drugs, 184
  and Secondary symptoms, 38
Principles and Organizations, 5
"Principles not Precedents," 123
Problems of homœopathy, 2
Process and products, 38
Provers, daybooks of, 155
Provings on the healthy, 242
Psora, 89, 99, 100, 102
  not a dyscrasia, 94
  and tuberculosis, identity of, 102
Purity of practice, 145

Q

Qualifications for practice, 2-4
Quantity and quality, 222, 242

R

Rabinowitsch, 103
Radiometer, 231

"Rational Medicine," 30
Raue, Chas. G., 161
Reaction, excessive, 85
Real cause, the logical, 268
Reappearance of suppressed symptoms, 121
Reasoning, modes of, 249, 252
Recall of the Medical Profession, 122
Reciprocal action, 10-13, 18
  law of, 174
Recoveries, mistaken for cures, 130
Relation, laws of, 222
Remedy, effect of the, 205-208
Repertories, 141, 263, 264
  work, generalizing for, 264
Repetition of doses, 202-205
Repulsion and attraction, 13, 14
Resistance, disease is, 62
  organic, 188
Responsibility, individual, 7
Rice, Philip, 113
"Rogue's Gallery," materia medica, 154
Rutherford on the atom, 230

S

Saboraud, 103
Science and art, relations of, 14
  definition of, 17
Science, Hahnemann's chief contribution to, 253
Sciences, relation of homœopathy to other, 15, 16
Sciolists, medical, 57
Scope of homœopathy, 37-47
"Scribes and Pharisees," 143
Second best remedy, 139, 140
Sequence of diseases, 12, 13
Serum and vaccine therapy, 55, 80
Shock, 82, 84, 85
Similia, sphere of, 42
Simple substance, 14
"Small doses," 183
Snyder, Carl, 217
Solutions, 228
Specialists and specialism, 48-50
Specialties, 169
Specifics for disease, 94, 241, 242
Spectrum analysis, 223
Spirit, the homœopathic, 3, 4
"Spiritual," Hahnemann's use of the word, 58
"Square Deal," the, 144
Stimulants and depressants, 82
"Subconscious pills," 143

Subjective symptoms, 150
Substantialism, 24, 26, 88
Substantialist, Hahnemann a, 26
Succession of phenomena, 266
Suggestion, therapeutic, 86
Suppressed diseases, 120
   symptoms, reappearance of, 121
Suppression of disease, 74
   evil results of, 133
Surgery, relation of, to medicine, 73
Susceptibility, 71, 76, 79, 81
   modification of, 194-202
   morbid, 121
   of the patient, 192
"Swat the Fly" campaign, 269
Swift, Dean, 101
Symptomatology, 147-166
Symptoms, aggravation of, 76, 116, 117, 152
   amelioration of, 153
   classification of, 172, 173
   defined, 39, 149
   general, 260
   negative-general, 26
   grading and grouping, 261
   memorizing, 262
   objective, 151
   particular, 261
   subjective, 150
   Totality of, 151-156
System, homœopathy a, 2

T

Talmud, 100
Terminal conditions, 196, 199
Therapeutic Idea, the, 153
   law, anticipations of, 252
Therapeutics, trend of modern, 132
"Thing itself," the, 33
Thompson, Prof. J. J., 235
Thompson, Wm. Gilman, 143
Thought, limitations of, 33
Totality of the symptoms, 38, 151-156
Totality, the diagnostic, 153
   logical, 255, 256
   numerical, 154
   therapeutic, 153

Toxicological theory of disease, 105-111
Treatment, basis of, 129
   object of, 129
Truth, opposition to, 1
Tubercular diseases, 103
Tuberculosis and Psora, 102
Two-fold existence of homœopathy, 2, 6

U

Unity of medicine, 48-59
Unity, pathological, 254

V

Vaccination, 219
Vaccines and serums, 219, 220
Vaccine treatment, 93
Valentin, 224
Validity of the homœopathic law, 4
Venereal diseases, 89, 90
Virchow, 66, 67
Vital activities, origin of, 61
   dynamics, 39, 40, 41
   Force, 64, 272
   Principle, 34, 88

W

"War of the Worlds," 6
Wells, P. P., 84, 161, 162, 176
Wesselhoeft, Conrad, 119
Wilkinson, J. J. Garth, 78, 213
Will, all force is, 63
Wood, Prof. J. C., 82
Working principles, Hahnemann's, 30

Z

Zeemann, on light, 230